HOMOLOGOUS ARTIFICIAL INSEMINATION (AIH)

CLINICS IN ANDROLOGY

E.S.E. HAFEZ, *series editor*

VOLUME 1

2. L.I. Lipshultz, J.N. Corriere Jr., E.S.E. Hafez, eds., Surgery of the male reproductive tract, 1980. ISBN 90-247-2315-9.
3. E.S.E. Hafez, ed., Descended and cryptorchid testis. 1980. ISBN 90-247-2299-3.
4. J. Bain, E.S.E Hafez, eds., Diagnosis in andrology. 1980. ISBN 90-247-2365-5.
5. G.R. Cunningham, W.-B. Schill, E.S.E. Hafez, eds., Regulation of male fertility. 1980. ISBN 90-247-2373-6.

series ISBN 90-247-2333-7

HOMOLOGOUS ARTIFICIAL INSEMINATION (AIH)

edited by

J.C. EMPERAIRE
Bordeaux, France

A. AUDEBERT
Bordeaux, France

and

E.S.E. HAFEZ
Detroit, Michigan, USA

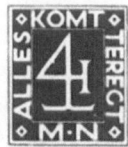

1980
MARTINUS NIJHOFF PUBLISHERS
THE HAGUE/BOSTON/LONDON

Distributors:

for the United States and Canada

Kluwer Boston, Inc.
160 Old Derby Street
Hingham, MA 02043
USA

for all other countries

Kluwer Academic Publishers Group
Distribution Center
P.O. Box 322
3300 AH Dordrecht
The Netherlands

Library of Congress Cataloging in Publication Data   CIP

Main entry under title:

Homologous artificial insemination (AIH)

   (Clinics in andrology; v. 1)
   Includes index.
   1. Artificial insemination, Human.
I. Emperaire, J.C.   II. Audebert, A.   III. Hafez, E.S.E., 1922-   IV. Series.
RG134.H65   618.1'7   79-26362

ISBN-13:978-94-009-8819-4   e-ISBN-13:978-94-009-8817-0
DOI: 10.1007/978-94-009-8817-0

TABLE OF CONTENTS

CONTRIBUTORS

AMIRIKIA, H.: Department of Gynecology and Obstetrics, Wayne State University School of Medicine, Detroit, Michigan 48201, USA

ANSARI, A.: Atlanta Fertility Institute, Baptist Professional Building, Suite 127, 340 Boulevard, N.E. Atlanta, Georgia 30312, USA

AUDEBERT, A.: Institut Aquitain de Recherches et d'Études de la Reproduction Humaine 40, cours de Verdun, 33000 Bordeaux, France

BARKAY, J.: Fertility Clinic, Department of Obstetrics and Gynecology, Central Emek Hospital, Afula, Israel

BARWIN, B.N.: Department of Obstetrics/Gynecology, Faculty of Medicine, University of Ottawa, 43 Bruyère, Ottawa K1N 9A9, Canada

BELAISCH, J.: 36, rue de Tocqueville, 75017 Paris, France

BERGER, M.J.: Department of Obstetrics and Gynecology, Harvard Medical School and Beth Israel Hospital, 330 Brookline Avenue, Boston, Massachusetts 02215 USA

BOLCIONI-AUTARD, A.M.: Centre des Problèmes de Reproduction et de Sexualité Humaines, 165 rue Saint-Pierre, 13005 Marseille, France

BOOKER, J.H.: Attorney-at-Law, 3101 North Woodward Aveneu, Suite 400, Royal Oak, Michigan 48072, USA

BOUHABEN-SITRI, M.C.: Centre des Problèmes de Reproduction et de Sexualité Humaines, 165 rue Saint-Pierre, 13005 Marseille, France

BROER, K.H.: University of Cologne Department of Obstetrics/Gynecology, Kerpenerstrasse 5, 5 Köln 41, Fed.Rep.Germany

CARRUTHERS, G.B.: 17 Harley Street, London W1, England

COHEN, J.: Clinique Marignan, 3 rue Marignan, Paris, France

COMHAIRE, F.: Department of Internal Medicine, Academisch Ziekenhuis, 135 de Pintelaan, B9000 Gent, Belgium

DEMPSEY, A: Department of Obstetrics/Gynecology, Faculty of Medicine, University of Ottawa, 43 Bruyère, Ottawa K1N 9A9, Canada

DMOWSKI, W.P.: Department of Obstetrics and Gynecology, Michael Reese Hospital and Medical Center, 29th Street and Ellis Avenue, Chicago, Illinois 60616, USA

EMPERAIRE, J.C.: Institut Aquitain de Recherches et d'Études de la Reproduction Humaines, 40 cours de Verdun, 33000 Bordeaux, France

ERICSSON, R.B.: Gametrics Ltd., 180 Harbor Drive, Sausality, California 94965, USA

FARI, A.: 5, boulevard de Strasbourg, 75010 Paris, France

FINEGOLD, W.J.: 4940 Bayard Street, Pittsburgh, Pennsylvania 15213, USA

GASSER, G.: Department of Urology and Ludwig Boltzmann Institute for Andrology, Krankenhaus der Stadt Wien-Lainz, Wolkerbergenstrasse 1, 1130 Vienna, Austria

GAYNOR, L.: Michael Reese Hospital and Medical Center, Pritzker School of Medicine, University of Chicago, Chicago, Illinois 60616, USA

HAAS, E.E.: Department of Obstetrics/Gynecology, Harvard Medical School and Beth Israel Hospital, 330 Brookline Avenue, Boston, Massachusetts 02215, USA

HAFEZ, E.S.E.: Department of Gynecology/Obstetrics and Andrology Research Unit, and C.S. Mott Center for Human Growth and Development, Wayne State University School of Medicine, Detroit, Michigan 48201, USA

HARRISON, R.: Department of Obstetrics/Gynaecology, University of Dublin, Trinity College Unit, Rotunda Hospital, Dublin, Ireland

JOLLY, E.E.: Department of Obstetrics/Gynecology, Faculty of Medicine, University of Ottawa, 43 Bruyère, Ottawa, K1N 9A9, Canada

KAPETANAKIS, E.: Michael Reese Hospital and Medical Center, Pritzker School of Medicine, University of Chicago, Chicago, Illinois 60616, USA

KREMER, J.: Fertility Unit, Department of Obstetrics & Gynecology, University Hospital, Utrecht, The Netherlands

LAWRENCE, M.: Michael Reese Hospital and Medical Center, Pritzker School of Medicine, University of Chicago, Chicago, Illinois 60616, USA

MATTEI, A.: Centre des Problèmes de Reproduction et de Sexualité Humaines, 165 rue Saint-Pierre, 13005 Marseille, France

McKAY, D.: Department of Obstetrics/Gynecology, Faculty of Medicine, University of Ottawa, 43 Bruyère, Ottawa K1N 9A9, Canada

NOOYER, DE C.A.A.: Department of Obstetrics/Gynecology, St. Elisabeth's of Groote Gasthuis, P.O. Box 417, 2000 AK Haarlem, The Netherlands

OS, W.A.A. VAN: St. Elisabeth's of Groote Gasthuis, P.O. Box 417, 2000 AK Haarlem, The Netherlands

PAULSON, J.: 1811 Ball Mill Court, Dunwoody, Georgia 30338, USA

PROPPING, S.: Department of OB/GYN, University Hospital, School of Medicine, Hufelandstrasse 55, 43 Essen, West Germany

RAO, R.: Michael Reese Hospital and Medical Center, Pritzker School of Medicine, University of Chicago, Chicago, Illinois 60616, USA

RHEMREV, P.E.R.: Department of Obstetrics/Gynecology, St. Elisabeth's of Groote Gasthuis, P.O. Box 417, 2000 AK Haarlem, The Netherlands

ROULIER, R.: Centre des Problèmes de Reproduction et de Sexualité Humaines, 165 rue Saint-Pierre, 13005 Marseille, France

SCHILL, W.B.: Dermatologische Klinik u. Poliklinik d. Universität, Frauenlobstrasse 9, 8 München 2, Fed.Rep.Germany

SCOMMEGNA, A.: Michael Reese Hospital and Medical Center, Pritzker School of Medicine, University of Chicago, Chicago, Illinois 60616, USA

SHERMAN, J.K.: Department of Anatomy, University of Arkansas Medical Sciences, Slot 510, 4301 W. Markham, Little Rock, Arkansas 72201 USA

STEENO, O.: Academisch Ziekenhuis, Sint-Rafael, Kapucijnenvoer 33, 3000 Leuven, Belgium

TAMOR, M.L.: Division of Infertility and Reproductive Endocrinology, Department of Obstetrics and Gynecology, Harvard Medical School and Beth Israel Hospital, 330 Brookline Avenue, Boston, Massachusetts 02215, USA

TIGNOL, J.: Clinique U.E.R. de Psychiatrie, 121 rue de la Bechade, 33076 Bordeaux Cedex, France

FOREWORD

Andrology, a counterpart to gynecology, deals with the study of the male reproductive organs. Clinical andrology has been neglected primarily because of the lack of relevant, accurate laboratory methods for functional analysis, but in the last decade substantial progress has been made in the understanding of male reproductive biology. This progress has resulted from modern techniques and instrumentation in microanatomy, immunology, neurophysiology, pathology, genetics, endocrinology, biochemistry, biophysics, urology and surgery. These studies are scattered in such a wide spectrum of journals that andrologists can hardly keep abreast of the advances. There have been numerous textbooks on the testes, male accessory organs and semen but the clinical aspects of andrology have not received similar emphasis. Since literature concerning clinical andrology is extensive and widely scattered in many different publications, we hope that a useful purpose will be served by summarizing the more pertinent material in a series of volumes which can be made readily available to students of andrology. It was decided that a series of specialized monographs should be devoted to clinics in andrology. These ten volumes of the series are an attempt to coordinate anatomical, physiological, biochemical, endocrinological, pharmacological and immunological aspects of the spermatozoa, testes, epididymis and other accessory genital organs. Little is known about the effect of diet, diseases, environmental factors and drugs on male reproduction. The interest in developing new male contraceptive methods will stimulate research in andrology. Some of these monographs present the results of several international conferences and symposia including those held in Bordeaux in May 1978; and the Pan American Congress of Andrology (PANCA), held in Caracas in March 1979.

Clinics in Andrology is intended to encourage the development of basic and clinical research in andrology, to analyze modern techniques for the evaluation of male reproduction, to recommend guidelines for therapeutic procedures, to standardize nomenclature, to recommend common norms of measurement, to promote an interchange of information and to stimulate the interest of scientists and clinicians in andrological problems.

Those who have provided illustrations have contributed greatly to the completion of this series and we hope that they feel that their material has been well used. It is our hope that this series will serve as a stimulus to basic scientists and clinicians concerned with andrology to intensify their research for better therapy of human ills. The editors wish to thank the contributors, who prepared their chapters meticulously, and Mr. Jeffrey Smith of Martinus Nijhoff for his fine cooperation during the production of this series.

E.S.E. Hafez
Detroit, Michigan,
USA

HOMOLOGOUS ARTIFICIAL INSEMINATION (AIH)

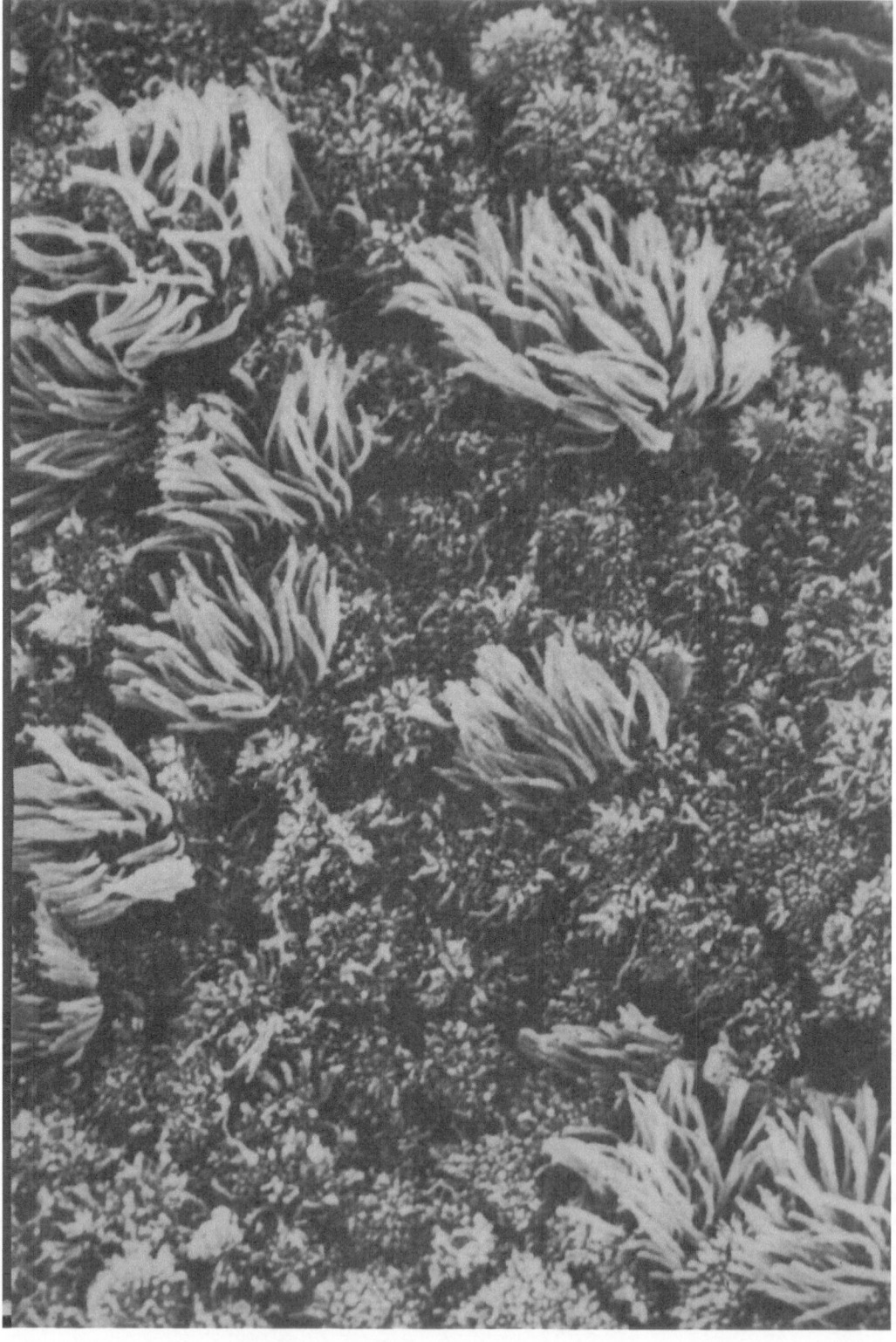

I. THE FEMALE PARTNER

1. EVALUATION OF THE FEMALE FERTILITY

J.C. EMPERAIRE and A. AUDEBERT

Male fertility is a relative notion, as it can only be expressed through a female partner, who herself is endowed with her own fertility. Female fertility, which is of great importance when dealing with infertility of the couple associated with male subfertility, becomes critical when AIH is considered, for at least two main reasons:

1. A significant number of pregnancies are associated with sperm parameters considered as low. Sperm concentration is reported as lower than 20 million spermatozoa per ml in as many as 5% of fertile couples (Mac Leod and Gold 1951; Rehan et al. 1975) and sperm motility inferior to 10% in as many as 10% of fertile couples (Page and Houlding 1951). Male subfertility may be masked by an excellent female fertility, as demonstrated by spermiograms taken prior to vasectomy in fertile couples (Smith et al. 1978). Aside from the possible intervention of another male partner, pregnancies associated with subfertile semen can only occur through prolonged exposure and/or a very high female fertility. The latter possibility seems to be supported by the percentage of fertile couples with subfertile semen, which may have increased in the past 25 years, possibly through a better evaluation and management of female causes of hypo-fertility (Zuckerman et al. 1977).

2. Artificial insemination with donor semen (AID), a situation where a normal sperm has replaced the supposed causative factor of infertility, is associated with a high failure rate. The overall pregnancy rate, either with fresh or frozen sperm, ranges from 35 to 45% in most recent comprehensive surveys (Friedman 1977; Sulewski et al. 1978). Accordingly, at least half of the patients engaged in AID procedures will not conceive despite an adequate sperm concentration, motility and morphology. Most reports on AID emphasize the role of female fertility in the pregnancy rate; this rate drops to 20% when an associated female subfertility factor is involved (Friedman 1977). On the other hand, another 22% is obtained after correction of pelvic disease (Sulewski et al. 1978) and the pregnancy rate may reach 67% after elimination of those women with associated causes of subfertility (Friedman 1977). The pregnancy rate is also higher in women with demonstrated fertility (Dixon and Buttram, 1976).

Considering these two points, the situation can only be worse when husband

artificial insemination (AIH) is considered, for (1) the parameters of the inseminated sperm, even after artificial improvement, are obviously lower than in
AID procedures; and (2) the percentage of highly fertile females is lower than in
the general population, as most of them would already have conceived despite a
subfertile semen.

   An acceptable rate of success with AIH can only be obtained through (1)
accurate inductions; (2) adequate amelioration of semen properties using split
ejaculation, filtration or in vitro treatment; and (3) improvement of the fertility
of the wife. Thus, a thorough evaluation must be conducted at the three critical
points of possible fertility defect, i.e. the cervical factor, the endocrine profile,
and the utero-adnexal function.

1. THE CERVICAL FACTOR

The cervical mucus acts as a reservoir for a continuous release of spermatozoa
towards the upper female genital tract (Hafez 1975). Optimal mucus properties
are required for an adequate sperm penetration and survival. A true cervical
cause is involved in 10 to 30% of infertility cases (Scott et al. 1977; Steinberg
1958). However, a mucus considered as subnormal, unable to interfere with a
normal sperm, may impair the progress of a subfertile semen.

   The penetrability of the cervical mucus is maximal during the late follicular
phase; maximal ferning, quantity and spinnbarkeit are associated 24 to 48 hours
before the shift in basal body temperature, BBT (Moghissi 1966). During other
periods of the menstrual cycle, the mucus is scanty, thick and readily immobilizes
sperm reaching the cervix. These cyclic changes are under hormonal control, and
the increased midcycle secretion of low-viscosity mucus is related to the preovulatory surge of estrogen production (Wolf et al. 1977a, 1977b).

   When dealing with male subfertility, the different types of postcoital tests are
of little value. The cervical factor must be assessed through the in vitro characteristics and penetrability of the cervical mucus.

1.1. The properties of the cervical mucus

Numerous reports have thoroughly analyzed the physical, chemical and ultrastructural properties and modifications of the cervical mucus along the menstrual
cycle (Wolf et al. 1977a, 1977b; Moghissi et al. 1960; Schumacher 1970; Hafez
1973). However, only a few physical characteristics are readily available to the
physician, and a clinical evaluation of the cervical secretions usually involves
macroscopic (abundance, transparency, stretchability) as well as microscopic
(cellularity, crystallization) information. No precise quantitative criteria are
available, because of (1) the difficulty of manipulating a hydrogel, and (2) the

highly variable pattern of spinnbarkeit and ferning among ovulating women. However, this pattern seems reproducible in the same patient (Blasco 1977). This evaluation remains mostly subjective, and a cervical score has been proposed (Insler and Melmed 1972).

When sampling the cervical mucus, the degree of opening of the cervical os must be recorded, and the cervix carefully checked for possible endo- and/or exocervicitis, or easy bleeding during manipulations. The mucus is taken from the endocervix either by gentle aspiration through a tuberculine syringe or with an atraumatic fenestrated forceps. The quantity and appearance of the mucus are noted; spinnbarkeit is roughly quantified by measuring the maximum length of stretchability of a thread of mucus between the two blades of the forceps. A mucus sample is deposited on a slide, checked for cellularity and then allowed to dry rapidly in open air to determine the ferning phenomenon. A normal pre-ovulatory mucus appears, flowing from an open cervical os, thin and watery; it may be easily stretched to 6-10 cm, and shows a massive ferning crystallization pattern.

The qualities of the cervical mucus are optimal during the few days prior to ovulation; conversely, the characteristics of the cervical mucus usually serve as a bases for the prediction of ovulation. Therefore, the assessment of the cervical factor is of little or no value if not supported by an accurate BBT chart.

Due to frequent ovulatory irregularities, a punctual observation of a low-quality mucus does not necessarily imply a cervical factor in female subfertility. In these cases, repeated evaluations must be carried out daily in the late follicular phase until the BBT shift suggests that ovulation has occurred.

1.2. In vitro penetration tests

Apparently satisfactory midcycle cervical mucus may be impenetrable to spermatozoa (Blasco et al. 1977). This underscores the lack of reliability of the readily available clinical criteria for cervical mucus quality. The performance of an in vitro penetration test prior to AIH procedures has been recommended by several authors (Kremer 1978; David et al. 1978), pointing out that the pregnancy rate is higher in the event of a satisfactory test.

The slide test, putting into contact a drop of mucus and a drop of semen with a coverslip, is not convenient for this purpose, as many physical factors appear to be involved (Moghissi et al. 1964). The best-suited in vitro procedure seems to be the capillary tube system, where an extremity of a capillary tube containing the mucus is plunged into a reservoir holding the sperm sample (Kremer 1965). The sperm penetration meter allows direct observation of the degree and distance of mucus penetration by spermatozoa.

Two requirements must be fulfilled for the test to be of any value:

- the cervical mucus must be apparently normal, either spontaneously or after synthetic estrogen therapy, as sperm does not penetrate thick and viscous samples (Kremer 1965, 1968);
- sperm motility must be subnormal, as only the spermatozoal movements are responsible for sperm penetration (Kremer 1965, 1968). The penetration test must be carried out with the husband semen sample which will be used in the AIH procedures: whole semen when normal, or treated semen – the better fraction of a split ejaculate, a sperm sample after glass wool or bovine serum albumine filtration, or semen after in vitro treatment (L. arginine, caffeine, kallicrein).

When a poor in vitro penetration test is associated with an apparently satisfactory cervical mucus and good motility in the sperm sample, in vitro crossed tests using both husband's and donor's semen, and wife's and donor's mucus must be carried out. They may point to an abnormal composition of the mucus (Blasco 1977), or to an immunological phenomenon (Franklin 1964).

Permanent low-quality mucus definitely points to an additional cervical factor of hypofertility, which has to be improved before AIH procedures are undertaken. Possible etiological factors (traumatic, infectious, or hormonal) must be thoroughly investigated and cured whenever possible. According to most reports, synthetic estrogen therapy at lower doses yields satisfactory results in 45% of cases of scanty or abnormal cervical mucus (Scott et al. 1977). The use of estrogens may, however, be ineffective at lower doses, but at higher, dosages they may disrupt the ovulatory pattern. In such cases we favour the use of human menopausal gonadotropins with hormonal monitoring, in an attempt the increase the endogenous level of estrogens.

When the defective cervical factor is not amenable to therapy, intrauterine insemination must be considered (Barwin 1974; White and Glass 1976). The conception rate appears higher in the presence of a satisfactory cervical mucus, as though the intrauterine insemination were in fact a retrograde intracervical insemination (Kremer 1978).

2. THE ENDOCRINE PROFILE

Most reproductive processes are under hormonal control, so various endocrine imbalances may reduce female fertility. This chapter will not deal with major disorders of the various endocrine tissues, as they have usually been diagnosed before the sterility problem has arisen. More discrete dysfunctions, however, may interfere with female reproduction, and these must be detected in the fertility assessment.

2.1. Thyroid function

Thyroid abnormalities have long been considered as the most classical cause of fertility disorders. However, the definition of accurate laboratory tests has permitted a critical reappraisal of this concept (Hamolsky 1975). Aside from gross thyroid diseases, most comprehensive reports tend to deny any significant responsibility of so-called 'mild hypothyroidism' in infertility (Tyler 1953; Schneeberg 1959). A complete fertility survey should nevertheless include a precise evaluation of the thyroid function, through protein-bound iodine and/ or free plasma T3 and T4 levels (Hamolsky 1975).

2.2. Androgenic function

Mild hyperandrogenism, from either adrenal or ovarian origin, may impair female fertility, which in turn is restored by corticosteroid suppression therapy (Greenblatt et al. 1956). A complete evaluation of the androgenic function includes the assay of plasma levels of testosterone, TEBG and delta-4 androstenedione. When these determinations are not readily available to the physician, an accurate evaluation of the fractioned urinary 17KS is of value for screening such patients (Emperaire and Blaizot 1978).

2.3. Luteal function

An inadequate corpus luteum remains a controversial putative cause of female subfertility. There is growing evidence, however, that a luteal phase defect may interfere with conception, egg transport and/or implantation and may be involved in about 3.5% of fertility problems (Jones 1975).

The low production of progesterone by an inadequate corpus luteum seems in turn to be related to abnormal FSH and LH secretion patterns during the follicular phase and/or the preovulatory period (Strott et al. 1970). The luteal phase defect may also result from other endocrine disorders, such as hypothyreosis, high plasma levels of androgens or mild hyperprolactinemia without menstrual disorders or galactorrhea (Lehmann and Bettendorf 1977). It may also be induced by various therapeutic agents, such as clomiphene citrate (Jones and Madrigal-Castro 1970).

There are no indisputable criteria for the diagnosis of luteal phase defect, which rather arises from the convergence of several indications.

The BBT chart, for instance, is a crude method for evaluation of luteal function, because it has an all or none type of response, and may be tampered with by patient inabilities. It may however point to a defective luteal phase, mostly in the case of the so-called short luteal phase, with a hyperthermic plateau of less than 9-11 days duration. On the other hand, the BBT curve may be apparently normal in the presence of a true luteal defect (Jones 1975).

The endometrial biopsy has represented until recently the most secure evaluation for luteal function. With the day of BBT shift and the day of the onset of following menses as points of reference, a lag of two days or more between the chronological and the endometrial dating is usually considered as indicative of luteal phase inadequacy (Jones 1975). In spite of the sometimes difficult determination of the exact day of ovulation on a BBT chart, the accuracy of the endometrial biopsy has recently been supported by the detection of the midcycle LH peak (Konincks et al. 1977). Although this histological proof may be difficult to establish, endometrial biopsy measures the target tissue response and represents a true bioassay for progesterone.

The determination of 24-hour urinary excretion of estrogens and pregnandiol after corpus luteum stimulation with HCG, together with adrenal suppression with dexamethazone, has been proposed ((Jayle 1956). This test may point to an estrogen deficiency, a progesterone deficiency, or both. The evaluation of serum progesterone reflects the functional state of the corpus luteum; however, daily determinations are not available for routine clinical assessment, and a single determination is not valid, due to day-to-day fluctuations.

The range of values for normal and abnormal function of the corpus luteum is still a matter of debate. Plasma progesterone values of 3 to 3.5 ng/ml seem sufficient for a BBT shift and a secretory endometrium (Israel et al. 1972). However, values around 5 ng/ml between days 4 and 11 postovulatory have been considered as the lower limit for the existence of functioning corpus luteum (Abraham et al. 1971). For others, a plasma progesterone level of 10 ng/ml is the boundary between normal corpus luteum function and luteal phase defect (Johansson 1969).

A single and well-timed serum progesterone determination has recently been favoured over a single endometrial biopsy for evaluation of luteal function (Shepard and Sentura 1977). However, the respective values of both explorations are still controversial, and both data should be obtained whenever possible for a correlated evaluation. Furthermore, due to the variability between successive cycles, the criteria for luteal phase inadequacy must be consistent on two consecutive cycles to be valid.

3. UTERINE FACTORS

Abnormalities of the uterine corpus are usually responsible for pregnancy complications or repeated miscarriages. They may however (1) interfere with the normal events leading to implantation, thus impairing female fertility, and (2) make difficult or hazardous the procedures of artificial insemination, especially when intrauterine. Past history and a careful clinical examination usually lead to the suspicion or the diagnosis of most uterine lesions, however an accurate evaluation requires various procedures.

Hysterography is the essential investigation which will serve as a basis for the assessment and the treatment of various lesions such as uterine hypoplasia or malformation, submucous leiomyoma, intrauterine adhesions, or endometrial polyps.

Hysteroscopy is a well-suited procedure for the treatment of intrauterine adhesions or the removal of small myomas. However it does not show any advantage over hysterography for diagnosis purposes, as an accurate radiographic study of the uterine cavity will recognize most uterine abnormalities.

Endometrial biopsy, beside its value in the hormonal evaluation, may discover a chronic endometritis causing a hostile uterine environment.

When a patient is at the point of considering AIH, hysterography and endometrial biopsy have usually already been performed at the beginning of the fertility survey of the couple. The detectable uterine factors have been discovered or ruled out.

4. TUBAL AND PERITONEAL FACTORS

Tubal factors are a major cause of female infertility; they may be involved in as many as 50% of the infertile couples. This high frequency accounts for the occasional association of tubal factors with another cause responsible for infertility. Thus a male hypofertility leading to AIH and appearing as the main cause of infertility does not exclude an associated tubal factor; conversely, tubal occlusions are not infrequently associated with various grades of male hypofertility.

A woman scheduled for AIH has undergone several basic infertility investigations, including the Rubin test and a hysterosalpingogram, which have concluded upon a presumed normal tubal function. However, if some tubal lesions may be predicted on the basis of previous history and physical examination, or easily detected by the above two investigations, some others will require a pelvic visualization to be recognized. Thus the Rubin test (mainly used for screening purposes) and salpingogram (despite a good visualization of the oviductal lumen) are both insufficient to rule out an abnormality of the tubal function, which process requires laparoscopy or culdoscopy.

When carefully performed and correctly interpreted, the findings of salpingography and laparoscopy are in disagreement in 40% of cases (Gomel 1977; Maathuis et al. 1972; Swolin and Rosencrantz 1972; and Keirse and Vandervellen 1973).

Radiologic investigations may be at fault in case of peritubal adhesions or partial occlusion of the fimbria, such as phimosis, which impairs oviductal mobility or passage. Pelvic visualization by endoscopy will allow an accurate evaluation. Laparoscopy will also detect unsuspected lesions, such as phimosis, peritubal adhesions and endometriosis, impairing fertility in about 50% of the cases of so-called 'unexplained sterility' in the apparently normal female partner (Peterson and Behrman 1970, Drake et al. 1977).

Laparoscopy is an irreplaceable investigation for infertility assessment; however, despite careful and correct indications, any endoscopy requires a general anesthesia, which has some unavoidable risks, even though rare. The timing of laparoscopy is a matter of debate: when any doubt on tubal function arises in the light of previous history, pelvic examination or salpingography, laparoscopy is mandatory prior to AIH. Endoscopy cannot be recommended routinely at this stage; in other instances, however, laparoscopy is again mandatory when AIH has been unsuccessfully performed for 4 to 6 cycles with no apparent reason accounting for these failures, as almost all pregnancies through AIH are recorded in the first 4 to 6 insemination cycles (Cohen and Delafontaine 1978; Finegold 1978; Keswani 1978). In such patients, pelvic visualization may discover lesions similar to those 'unexplained sterility' in up to 60% of the women (Mintz 1978), leading to various specific treatments (lysis of adhesions, fimbrioplasty or medical treatment of endometriosis).

Figure 1 shows a tentative diagram for the survey of female fertility when AIH is considered.

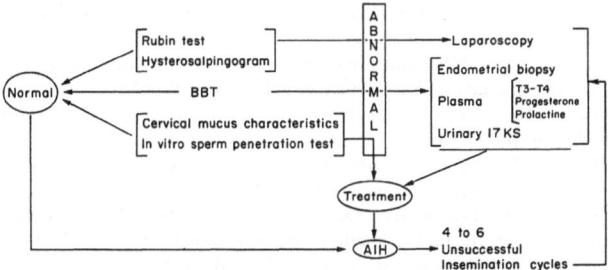

REFERENCES

Abraham GE, Swerdloff R, Tulchinsky D, Odell WD: Radioimmunoassay of plasma progesterone. *J Clin Endocrin Metab* 32:619, 1971.
Barwin BN: Intrauterine insemination of husband's semen. *J Reprod Fertil* 36:101, 1974.
Blasco L: Clinical approach to the evaluation of sperm cervical mucus interactions. *Fertil Steril* 28(11):1133, 1977.
Blasco L, Sokoloski J, Wolf DP: Factors which affect sperm penetrability in human cervical mucus: abstract. *Fertil Steril* 28:308, 1977.
Cohen J, Delafontaine D: AIH with split ejaculate for male subfertility. Presented at the first international symposium on AIH and male subfertility, Bordeaux, 1978.

David G, Gernigon C, Kunstmann JM: Insémination artificielle avec sperme du conjoint. *J Gyn Obst Biol Repr* 16(7):686, 1978.

Dixon RE, Buttram VC: Artificial insemination using donor semen: a review of 171 cases. *Fertil Steril* 27(2):130, 1976.

Drake T, Tredway D, Buchanan G, Takaki N: Unexplained infertility: a reappraisal. *Obstet Gynec.* 50:644-646, 1977.

Emperaire JC, Blaizot O: Métabolisme et action physiologique des hormones mâles. *Rev Médecine* 31(19):1709, 1978.

Finegold WJ: Artificial insemination homologous. Presented at the first international symposium on AIH and male subfertility, Bordeaux, 1978.

Franklin R, Dukes CD: Anti-spermatozoal antibody and unexplained infertility. *Am J Obstet Gynecol* 89:6, 1964.

Friedman S: Artificial donor insemination with frozen human semen. *Fertil Steril* 28(11):1230, 1977.

Gomel V: Laparoscopy prior to reconstructive tubal surgery for infertility. *J Reprod Med* 18:251-253, 1977.

Greenblatt RB, Barfield WE, Lampros CP: Cortisone in the treatment of infertility. *Fertil Steril* 7:203, 1956.

Hafez ESE: Transport of spermatozoa in the female reproductive tract. *Am J Obstet Gynecol* 115:703, 1973.

Hafez ESE: Sperm transport. In: *Progress in infertility*, Behrman SJ, Kistner RW (eds.). Boston, Little, Brown, 1975 (2nd ed.).

Hamolsky MW: Thyroid factors. In *Progress in infertility*. Behrman SJ, Kistner RW (eds.), Boston, Little, Brown, 1975 (2nd ed.).

Insler VH, Melmed I: The cervical score. *Int J Gyn Obst* 10:223, 1972.

Israel R, Mishell DR, Stone SC, Thorneycroft IH, Moyer DL: Single luteal phase serum progesterone assay as an indication of ovulation. *Am J Obstet Gynecol* 112:1043, 1972.

Jayle MF: Exploration biochimique du corps jaune. *Gynecol Prat* 7:3, 1956.

Johansson EDB: Progesterone levels in peripheral plasma during the luteal phase of the normal human menstrual cycle measured by a rapid competitive protein-binding technique. *Acta Endocr (KBH)* 61:592, 1969.

Jones GS: Luteal phase defects. In: *Progress in infertility*, Behrman SJ, Kistner RW (eds.), Boston, Little, Brown, 1975, p. 299.

Jones GS, Madrigal-Castro V: Hormonal findings in association with abnormal corpus luteum function in the human: the luteal phase defect. *Fertil Steril* 21:1, 1970.

Keirse MJ, Vandervellen R: A comparison of hysterosalpingography and laparoscopy in the investigation of infertility. *Obstet Gynecol* 14:685-688, 1973.

Keswani SG: AIH for subfertility with frozen and fresh sperm concentrates. Presented at the first international symposium on AIH and male subfertility, Bordeaux, 1978.

Konincks PR, Goddeeris PG, Lauweryns JM, Hertog RC, Brosens IA: Accuracy of endometrial biopsy dating in relation to the midcycle luteinizing hormone peak. *Fertil Steril* 28(4):443, 1977.

Kremer J: A simple sperm penetration test. *Int J Fertil* 10:201, 1965.

Kremer J: The in vitro spermatozoal penetration test in fertility investigations. Thesis, Groningen, The Netherlands, 1968.

Kremer J: In vitro sperm penetration in cervical mucus and AIH. Presented at the first international symposium on AIH and male subfertility, Bordeaux, 1978.

Lehmann F, Bettendorf G: Pathology of corpus luteum function and its treatment. *Fertil Steril* 28(3):291, 1977.

Maathuis JB, Horbach JGH, Mall EV van: A comparison of the results of hysterosalpingography and laparoscopy in the diagnosis of Fallopian tube dysfunction. *Fertil Steril* 23:428-431, 1972.

MacLeod J, Gold RZ: The male factor in fertility and infertility II: spermatozoon counts in 1000 cases of human fertility and in 1000 cases of infertile marriage. *J Urol* 66:436, 1951.

Mintz M: Laparoscopy and artificial insemination: indications and results. Presented at the first international symposium on AIH and male subfertility, Bordeaux, 1978.

Moghissi KS: Cyclic changes of cervical mucus in normal and progestin treated women. *Fertil Steril* 17:663, 1966.

Moghissi KS, Neuhaus OW, Stevenson CS: Composition and properties of human cervical mucus I: electrophoretic separation and identification of proteins. *J Clin Invest* 39:1358, 1960.

Moghissi KS, Darich D, Lebine J, Neuhans OW: Mechanism of sperm migration. *Fertil Steril* 15:15, 1964.

Page EN, Houlding F: The clinical interpretation of 1000 semen analyses among applicants for sterility studies. *Fertil Steril* 2:140, 1951.

Peterson EP, Behrman SJ: Laparoscopy of the infertile patient. *Obstet Gynecol* 35:363-367, 1970.

Rehan NE, Sobrero AJ, Fertig JW: The semen of fertile men: a statistical analysis of 1300 men. *Fertil Steril* 26(6):492, 1975.

Schneeberg NG: The thyroid gland and infertility. *Clin Obstet Gynecol* 2:286, 1959.

Schumacher GFB: Biochemistry of cervical mucus. *Fertil Steril* 21:697, 1970.

Scott JZ, Nakamura RM, Mutch J, Davajan V: The cervical factor in infertility: diagnosis and treatment. *Fertil Steril* 28(12):1289, 1977.

Shepard MK, Sentura YD: Comparison of serum progesterone and endometrial biopsy for confirmation of ovulation and evaluation of luteal function. *Fertil Steril* 28(5):541, 1977.

Smith KD, Stulz DR, Jackson RJ, Steinberger E: Evaluation of sperm counts and total sperm counts in 2543 men requesting vasectomy. *Andrologia* 10(5):362, 1978.

Soules MR, Wiebe RH, Aksel S, Hammond CB: The diagnosis and therapy of luteal phase deficiency. *Fertil Steril* 28(10):1033, 1977.

Steinberg N: The role of the cervical factor in sterility. *Fertil Steril* 9:407, 1958.

Strott CA, Cargille CM, Ross GT, Lipsett MB: The short luteal phase. *J Clin Endocrin Metab* 30:246, 1970.

Sulewski JM, Eisenberg MD, Stenger VG: A longitudinal analysis of artificial insemination with donor semen. *Fertil Steril* 29:527, 1978.

Swolin K, Rosencrantz M: Laparoscopy vs. hysterosalpingography in sterility investigations: a comparative study. *Fertil Steril* 23:270-273, 1972.

Tyler ET: The thyroid myth in infertility. *Fertil Steril* 4:218, 1953.

Wallach EE: The uterine factors in infertility. *Fertil Steril* 23:138-158, 1972.

White RM, Glass RH: Intrauterine insemination with husband's semen. *Obstet Gynecol* 47(1):119, 1976.

Wolf DP, Blasco L, Khan MA, Litt M: Human cervical mucus I: rheologic properties. *Fertil Steril* 28:41, 1977 (a).

Wolf DP, Blasco L, Khan MA, Litt M: Human cervical mucus II: changes in viscoelasticity during the ovulatory menstrual cycle. *Fertil Steril* 28:47, 1977 (b).

Zuckerman Z, Rodriguez-Rigau LJ, Smith KD, Steinberger E: Frequency distribution of sperm counts in fertile and infertile males. *Fertil Steril* 28(12):1310, 1977.

2. PHYSIOLOGY OF SPERMATOZOA INSEMINATED IN THE FEMALE REPRODUCTIVE TRACT

E.S.E. HAFEZ

The physicochemical and immunological factors in the vagina and cervix at the time of artificial insemination play an important role in sperm survival and transport into the uterus and oviduct. The vaginal secretions immobilize spermatozoa within one to two hours of insemination. The rapid elimination and immobilization of spermatozoa in the vagina make it essential for the rapid transport of sperm to a more favourable environment.

Seminal plasma plays a major role in the transport and the physiology of spermatozoa. However, spermatozoa from the vas deferens and epididymis are successfully used in artificial insemination, and removal of various accessory organs of the male tract rarely decreases fertility as long as ejaculation still results in the release of a few million spermatozoa through the urethra.

Unlike the vagina, the epithelial lining of the cervix, uterus, and oviduct is made of nonciliated secretory cells and kinociliated cells. In general, secretory cells have a dome-shaped surface covered with numerous microvilli, and their cytoplasm contains numerous secretory granules. The percentage of kinociliated cells in the epithelium, which varies in different parts of the reproductive tract, is maximal in the fimbriae and oviductal ampulla and minimal in the uterus and uterine cervix (Hafez 1972). The ciliated cells are covered with kinocilia which beat rhythmically toward the vagina.

1. SPERM DISTRIBUTION IN THE FEMALE REPRODUCTIVE TRACT

Three stages are recognized in sperm transport in the female reproductive tract (Figure 1, Table 1): rapid short sperm transport; colonization of reservoirs; and slow, prolonged release (Hafez 1975, 1976).

1.1. Rapid transport

Immediately after insemination, spermatozoa penetrate the micelles of the cervical mucus where some are quickly transported through the cervical canal. This phase takes from two to ten minutes and may be facilitated by increased contractile activity of the myometrium and mesosalpinx during courtship and

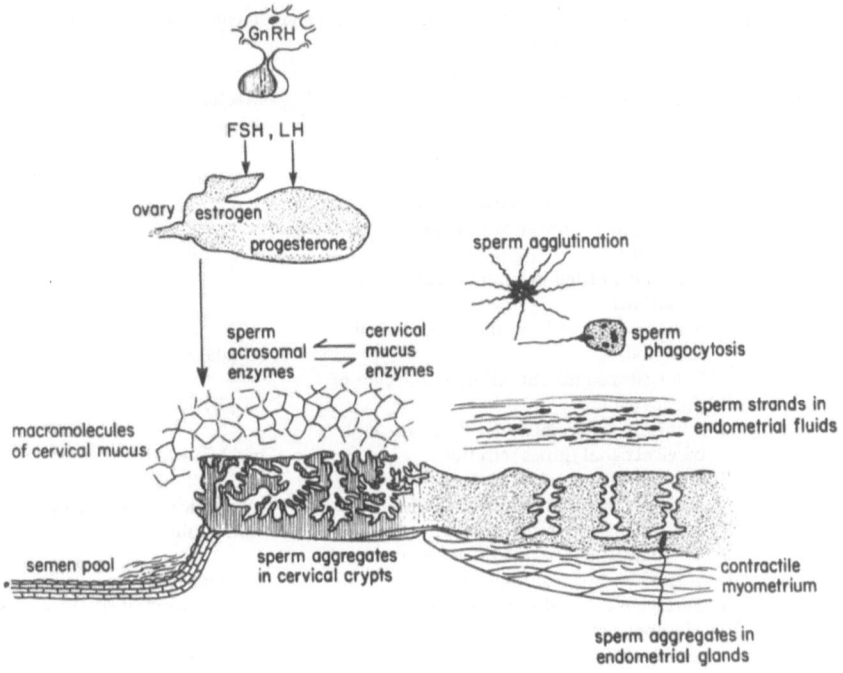

Figure 1. Diagrammatic illustration of the physiological and endocrine mechanisms of sperm transport in the female reproductive tract.

coitus. Some spermatozoa reach the internal os of the cervix within 1.5 to 3 minutes after insemination. Some sperm can thus reach the site of fertilization very rapidly. It is not known whether the first sperm entering the oviduct are those which participate in fertilization of the ovum, but it has been proposed that fertilization only occurs when a critical number of spermatozoa reach the site of fertilization.

1.2. Colonization of sperm reservoirs

Massive numbers of spermatozoa are trapped in the complex mucosal folds of the cervical crypts. This process is facilitated by the fact that the micelles of the cervical mucus help to direct spermatozoa to the cervical crypts where the reservoir is formed. Fewer leukocytes are found in the cervical secretions compared with those of the vagina or uterus. This suggests that less phagocytosis of spermatozoa takes place in the cervix. Concentration gradients of spermatozoa are established within a short time interval after intercourse. The more spermatozoa that enter the cervical reservoir the more will reach the oviduct, increasing the chance of fertilization. In addition, the larger the reservoir, the longer an

Table 1. Summary of sequence of events of major physiological phenomena associated with spermatozoa transport in the male and female reproductive tracts.

Site	Physiological phenomena	Mechanisms involved
Male reproductive tract	1. Spermatozoa undergo maturation in cauda epididymis	neuromuscular
	2. At ejaculation, spermatozoa released from epididymis are mixed with male accessory secretions	metabolic
	3. Semen deposited in several ejaculatory pulsations	
Vagina	4. Semen mixed with vaginal and cervical secretions	copulatory motor activities
Cervix	5. Spermatozoa migrate through micelles of cervical mucus	biophysical
	6. Abnormal spermatozoa filtered through cervical canal (gross selection)	biochemical
	7. Cervical crypts establish spermatozoa reservoir or reject excessive spermatozoa causing massive reduction in number	mechanical (kinocilia of epithelium)
Uterus	8. Spermatozoa separated from seminal plasma and transported to oviduct	myometrial contraction
	9. Surface plasma of spermatozoa removed	agglutination of spermatozoa
	10. Metabolic changes and capacitation of spermatozoa	biochemical
	11. Acrosomal proteinase (trypsin-like enzyme) inactivated by trypsin inhibitors from seminal plasma	leukocytes; enzymatic
Uterotubal junction	12. Quantitative selection of spermatozoa	mechanical
Isthmus	13. Spermatozoa numbers reduced	
	14. Control of egg transport in oviduct	neural
	15. Spermatozoa plasma membrane changes (acrosome reaction); spermatozoa capacitation	biochemical
Ampulla	16. Spermatozoa motility increases in oviductal fluid in order to penetrate corona radiata and zona pellucida	mechanical / metabolic
	17. Reduction division of gametes completed	enzymatic
	18. Acrosomal proteinase released	biophysical
	19. Selection at egg surface (receptors?) by spermatozoa	
Fimbriae	20. Excessive spermatozoa lost into peritoneal cavity	spermatozoa motility

adequate population of spermatozoa will be maintained in the oviduct. Spermatozoa may leave the cervix by their own motility or be passively transported by cervical and uterine contractions.

In species where ejaculation occurs in the uterine lumen, sperm reservoirs are localized in the uterotubal junction as in the pig or in the endometrial glands as in the dog. There is no evidence to show that spermatozoa are released after their entry into the endometrial glands of any species.

1.3. Slow release and transport

After adequate sperm reservoirs are established within the reproductive tract, the spermatozoa are released sequentially for a prolonged period. This slow release, which involves the innate motility of spermatozoa and contractile activity of the myometrium and mesosalpinx, ensures continued availability of spermatozoa for entry into the oviduct to effect fertilization of the egg.

2. SPERM TRANSPORT IN THE CERVIX

The endocervical mucosa (Figure 2, Figure 3) is an intricate system of clefts, grooves and crypts grouped together (Hafez 1973a, 1973b). The endocervical canal contains approximately 100 secretory units which secrete the cervical mucus into the lumen of the canal (Odeblad 1966). Several functions have been ascribed to the cervix and its secretion: (a) to provide receptivity to sperm penetration at or near ovulation and to inhibit migration at other phases of the cycle; (b) to act as a sperm reservoir; (c) to protect spermatozoa from the hostile environment of the vagina and from being phagocytized; (d) to provide spermatozoa with energy requirements; (e) to filter defective and immotile spermatozoa; and (f) possibly to participate in capacitation of spermatozoa (Moghissi 1973; Hafez and Thibault 1975).

2.1. Cervical mucus

Cervical mucus which accumulates in the vaginal pool may contain endometrial, oviductal, follicular, and peritoneal fluids as well as leukocytes and cellular debris from uterine, cervical, and vaginal epithelia. The endocervical crypts in women of reproductive age secrete 20 to 60 mg of mucus per day which increases to 700 mg per day during midcycle (Odeblad 1966). These secretions are hydrogels which consist of water and a solid component made of three or more units forming a three-dimensional network. The secretions are heterogenous in composition, due to two types of low and high-viscosity components (Odeblad 1959). The low-viscosity fraction, a yellowish fluid readily aspirated into a capillary tube, is composed of nonmucin proteins (characteristic of serum proteins), salts, lipids, and carbohydrates. The high-viscosity fraction, a clear, white, very viscous substance, contains mucins which are the glycoproteins or glycopeptides responsible for the gel formation (Odeblad 1968).

The midcycle cervical mucus is composed of macromolecules arranged into micellar units which are made up of some 100 to 1000 chains of macromolecules. The estimated diameter of each micellar unit is 1.5 microns. At various loci, the micelles give out side chains which connect them to neighboring micelles forming

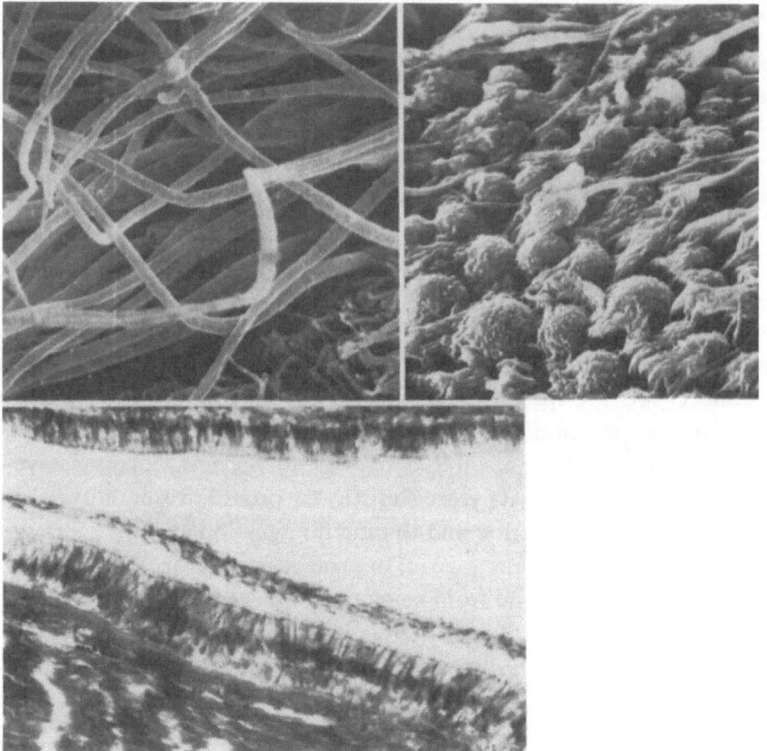

Figure 2. Scanning electron micrographs of spermatozoa and cervical tissue showing the relationship of spermatozoa motility to cilia beat and movement of mucus in the cervix uteri. Macromolecules of cervical mucus are arranged in filament-like micelles. During midcycle, active spermatozoa are transported through the channels of micelles against the direction of cilia beat. Intricate biophysical and biochemical relationships may exist between micelles of mucus, leukocytes, and spermatozoa. The cervical cilia are important for the directional flow of the cervical mucus from the narrow crypts to the cervical lumen. Upper left: note the alignment of spermatozoa in one direction in the lumen of the cervix (4,700 ×); *upper right:* note the heads of spermatozoa embedded in the kinocilia within the endocervix (2,000 ×) lower: within the uterus, note arrangement of spermatozoa in strands.

a honycomb-like network of macromolecules which is responsible for the macro-rheological properties of cervical mucus. Davajan et al. (1970) postulated that such a physical system allows a watery fluid (the low-viscosity component) to flow in a specific direction between 'rods' of high-viscosity mucus which are fixed within the secreting crypts. The macromolecules of mucins of cervical mucus have a polypeptide backbone with oligosaccharide and sialic acid side chains. Proteolytic hydrolysis of the mucus or its mucins by proteolytic enzymes causes physical and biochemical changes.

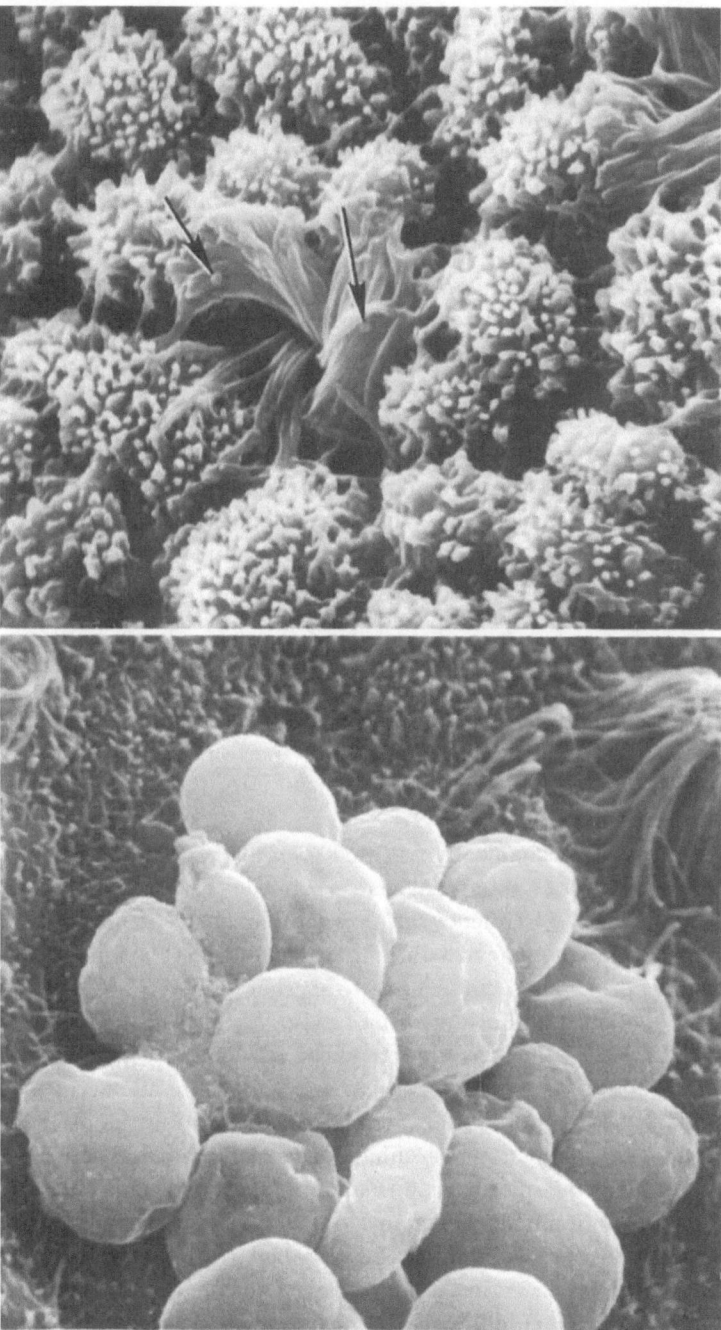

Figure 3. Top: secretory and ciliated cells (arrow) in the cervical mucus (3,200 ×); *bottom:* leukocytes found in the uterus noted 12 hours after intercourse (5,000 ×).

Cervical mucus has several rheological properties such as viscosity, flow elasticity, spinnbarkeit, thixotropy, and tack (stickiness). Low-molecular-weight organic components include free simple sugars (glucose, maltose, and mannose) and amino acids. The mucus also contains proteins, trace elements and enzymes (Schumacher 1970; Schumacher and Pearl 1968).

2.2. Sperm penetration in cervical mucus

Information on the cyclic changes of cervical mucus which may stimulate or inhibit sperm transport in the female reproductive tract is essential for a better understanding of problems of infertility and contraceptive research. It would thus be possible to develop a contraceptive method by which the watery, mid-cycle mucus can be safely altered to a viscous barrier to sperm transport without affecting the ovary-pituitary-hypothalamus interrelationships.

Sperm penetrability in the cervical mucus begins approximately on the ninth day of a normal menstrual cycle, increases gradually to a peak at ovulation, persists for two to seven days, and is inhibited until the following midcycle (Figure 4). Individual variances in the length of the period for sperm pene-trability are remarkable. Sperm penetrability increases with the cleanliness of the mucus, since cellular debris and leukocytes delay sperm migration.

Ejaculated spermatozoa rapidly penetrate watery cervical mucus during mid-cycle, aided principally by sperm motility as well as by the micro- and macro-rheological properties of mucus. The rate of sperm penetration in the mucus varies throughout the menstrual cycle from 0.1 to 3 mm per minute and is maximal in the ovulatory stage.

Spermatozoa are mechanically oriented toward the internal os. As the fla-gellum beats and vibrates, the sperm head is propelled forward in the channels of least resistance. The tail frequency sets up a mechanical resonance between itself and the oscillation frequency of the molecular lattice (Davajan et al. 1970). Hydrodynamic principles seem to apply to sperm motility; thus, motile sperma-tozoa are in dynamic equilibrium with the viscous force of the medium rather than being affected by the inertial force which influences large moving objects. In order to account for spermatozoa moving with minimal energy expended, Odeblad (1968) has proposed that there may be oscillations along the micelles (waves) in the cervical mucus which enhance sperm migration. These oscillations are associated with the microscopic filaments (macromolecular chains) in the flexible component of mucus (Davajan et al. 1970). It is possible that the beat of kinocilia in the endocervix maintains this so-called oscillation in cervical mucus.

India ink particles placed in the human cervical canal were recovered in the oviducts in 30% of cases (de Boer 1972). Dead pig spermatozoa inseminated in pigs were transported to the oviduct less efficiently than live spermatozoa (Baker and Degen 1972). It would appear that sperm mobility facilitates penetrability but is not absolutely necessary.

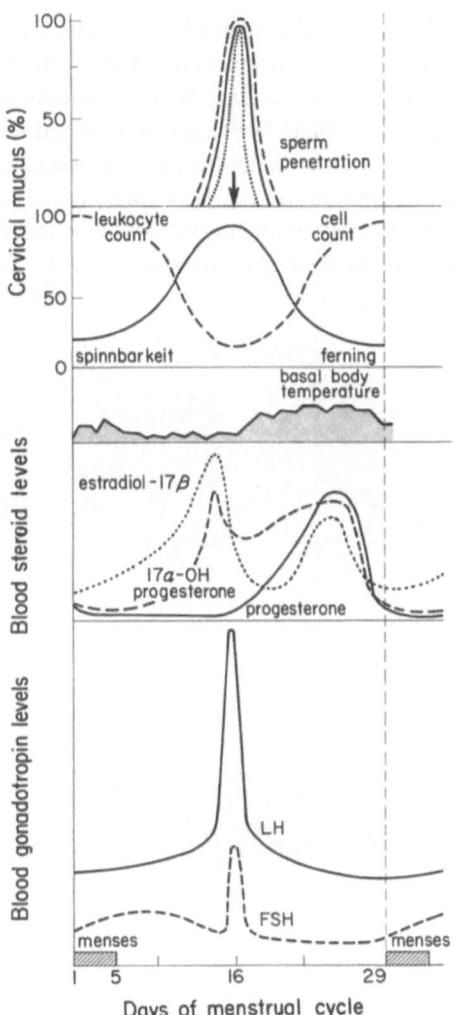

Figure 4. Cyclical changes in sperm penetration in cervical mucus as they relate to biophysical changes in cervical mucus and fluctuations in endocrine profile.

The aqueous spaces between the micelles allow the passage of sperm as well as the diffusion of soluble substances. Proteolytic enzymes (proteinases in seminal plasma) may hydrolyze the backbone protein or some of the cross-lineages of the mucin and thus reduce the network to a less resistant mesh with more open channels for the enhancement of sperm migration. It is also possible that the release of spermatozoa from the cervical crypts opposed by filaments of glyco-protein depends on hydrolysis of these chains by sperm head proteases.

Although spermatozoa appear to move at random in the cervical secretion

(Figure 5), they probably follow the path of least resistance along strands of cervical mucus. When migration of a spermatozoon in mucus is impeded, the sperm usually resumes its forward course with a sudden deflection into an adjacent parallel path (Kremer 1968). When semen is mixed with cervical mucus in vitro a sharp boundary occurs between the two fluids and the cervical mucus is penetrated by fingerlike phalanges. Phalanx formation may function to (a) increase surface area between semen and cervical mucus; (b) provide pockets of semen within the mucus, to protect spermatozoa from the hostile vaginal en-

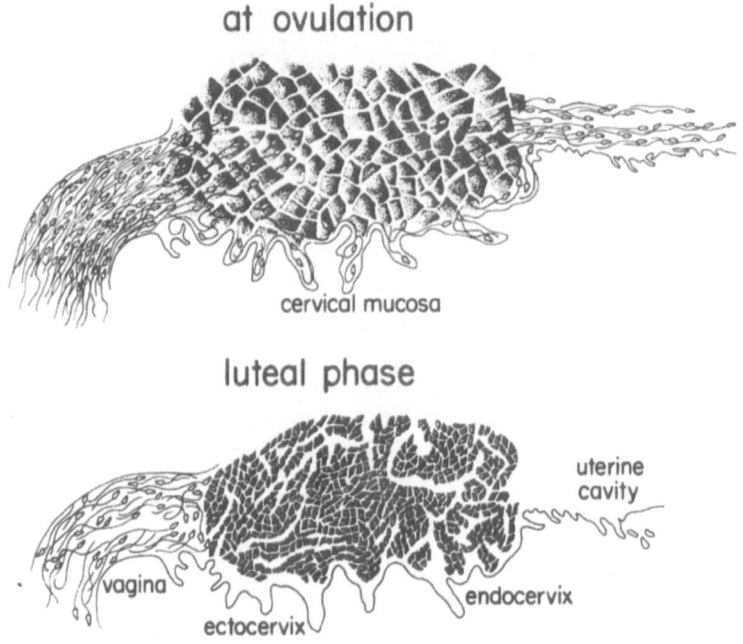

Figure 5. Changes in biophysical characteristics and dimensions of mesh in cervical mucus during luteal phase as compared to the time of ovulation.

vironment; and (c) facilitate sperm migration into the uterine cavity. Sperm phalanges develop significant degrees of arborization, the terminal aspects of which consist of canals through which only one or two spermatozoa can pass.

The rapid initial short transit time in the human cervix lasts 5-10 minutes after insemination, whereas more constant prolonged release of sperm to the upper genital tract occurs 10-150 minutes after insemination (Tredway et al. 1975). From 15 minutes after insemination, the number of sperm within the cervical mucus remains fairly constant until a definite decline is noted at 24 hours; and by 48 hours the number of sperm is negligible.

3. SPERM TRANSPORT IN THE UTERUS

Intrauterine postcoital samples show considerably fewer numbers of abnormal spermatozoa than the ejaculate. This may be due to the fact that only motile spermatozoa can penetrate cervical mucus. The contractile activity of the vagina and myometrium plays a major role in the transport of spermatozoa into and through the uterus. Combined postcoital tests and endometrial aspirations have shown that the maximal number of spermatozoa in the uterine lumen are found at, or near, ovulation. Very few spermatozoa were found in the uterus during the luteal or early follicular phases of the cycle (Frenkel 1961). Massive numbers of spermatozoa invade the endometrial glands. It is believed that the presence of spermatozoa in the uterus induces endometrial leukocytic response which enhances phagocytosis of excessive numbers of living and probably dead spermatozoa.

Early investigators believed that intercourse caused an increase in the muscular activity of the uterus – an inward-outward movement of the mucus column in the cervical canal with the subsequent 'sucking in' of semen – that facilitated sperm migration. Sperm transport was thus explained as a 'passive' phenomenon which was attributed to the negative pressure in the abdominal cavity of the female. It seems unlikely, however, that this negative pressure can be effectively transmitted to the lower reproductive tract to enhance uterine contraction and sperm transport. Sobrero (1967) fitted a group of women with a snug cervical cap containing a water-soluble opaque medium. Radiopaque fluid placed in the cervical cap did not enter the uterus after coitus or clitoral stimulation. Sexual stimulation also caused minimal dilation of the external os (Masters and Johnson 1966, p. 114). Also, the pregnancy rate is high following artificial insemination in which semen is deposited in the vagina or on the cervix in the absence of orgasm and seminal aspiration. Much more evidence supports 'active' transport which is attributed to the motility of spermatozoa aided by the realignment of micro- and macromolecules of cervical mucus.

4. TRANSPORT IN THE OVIDUCT

The oviduct has the unique function of conveying spermatozoa and eggs in opposite directions almost simultaneously. The pattern and rate of sperm transport through the oviduct are controlled by several mechanisms, such as peristalsis and antiperistalsis of oviductal musculature, complex contractions of the oviductal mucosal folds and of the mesosalpinx, fluid currents and countercurrents created by ciliary action, and possibly the opening and closing of the intramural portion. The relative importance of these mechanisms in sperm transport through the oviduct is unknown. Oviductal contractions alter the configuration of the oviductal compartments momentarily, so that fluids and suspending spermatozoa may be transported toward the fimbriae from one compartment to the next. In the oviduct of the pigeon and painted tortoise, there are two systems of kinocilia: one beats toward the ovary and the other toward the cloaca. These two ciliary systems are capable of moving particles in opposite directions.

Ahlgren (1969) studied sperm transport in three fertile and 177 infertile women. Patients were examined after intercourse or artificial insemination for the presence of sperm in the cervical mucus, the uterine cavity (by transcervical aspiration), and the oviducts (by laparoscopy or laparotomy). The number of spermatozoa in the cervical mucus and uterine cavity was highly correlated with that in the oviduct and pouch of Douglas. The maximal number of motile spermatozoa were noted in all segments in the presence of a mature follicle in the ovaries. In the presence of a corpus luteum, the number of motile spermatozoa decreased.

A few critical investigations have been carried out to estimate the optimum number of spermatozoa needed in the oviduct for normal fertilization. During the course of laparotomy or laparoscopy, Ahlgren (1971) flushed the oviducts of 49 infertile women 2-34 hours after coitus or artificial insemination, coitus being restricted to a period of at least four days before the 'admissional intercourse'.

5. ENDOCRINE CONTROL OF SPERM TRANSPORT

More is known about the endocrine control of ovulation and spermatogenesis than about endocrinology of sperm transport in the female tract. Ovarian hormones affect (a) the structure, ultrastructure, and secretory activity of the cervical, uterine, and oviductal epithelium; (b) the contractile activity of the uterotubal musculature; (c) the quantitative and qualitative characteristics of cervical mucus, and uterine and oviductal secretions. Changes are noted in the protein content, enzyme activity, electrolytes, surface tension, and conductivity of these fluids. Increasing the amount of endogenous estrogen during the preovulatory phase of the cycle or the administration of synthetic estrogens produces copious amounts of thin, watery, cervical secretions. Endogenous progesterone during the luteal phase of the cycle or in pregnancy produces scanty, viscous, cellular cervical mucus with low spinnbarkeit and ferning. The penetrability of spermatozoa is greatly inhibited in the progestational cervical mucus. It is possible that the cyclical changes in cervical mucus are mechanisms to protect the female from unnecessary exposure to the foreign proteins of semen.

Sperm transport in the female genital tract is also controlled by oxytocin, and the sympathetic and parasympathetic nervous systems. Epinephrine, acetylcholine, histamine, and various vasoconstrictors can alter uterine contraction but the effects are transient, and neither denervation of the uterus, transection of the spinal cord, nor reversal of a segment of the uterus completely inhibits sperm transport.

The human seminal plasma contains high concentrations of various prostaglandins secreted by the seminal vesicles. Most of the prostaglandins can influence the motility of the human myometrium and oviduct. The contraction of the myometrium is dependent on several factors but there is some evidence that the seminal prostaglandins may facilitate the passive sperm transport within the female genital tract. The sensitivity of the human uterus to prostaglandins reaches a peak between the late proliferative and early secretory phases of the menstrual cycle. Intravaginal application of seminal plasma or partially purified prostaglandins from semen influence the motility and tonus of both uterus and oviducts (Eliasson and Passe 1960). There is also an increase in the resistance to insufflation during Rubin's test within 25-40 minutes after vaginal application of prostaglandin.

6. SPERM TRANSPORT AND FERTILITY

The continuous flow of spermatozoa from the cervix is associated with phagocytosis of spermatozoa within the uterus, and loss of sperm into the peritoneal cavity. Thus, a population of fertilizable spermatozoa is being maintained at the site of fertilization near the ampullary isthmic junction of the oviduct. The percentage of morphologically normal spermatozoa is higher in the oviducts and uterus than in the ejaculate. Some morphologically abnormal spermatozoa may reach the oviduct, although to a lesser extent. Filtering of dead, abnormal and incompetent sperm during their passage through the reproductive tract ensures the greatest viability of the zygote. It is possible that ejaculates containing high concentrations of abnormal spermatozoa may be associated with a high rate of spontaneous abortion.

In men with faulty spermatogenesis it is possible that the minimum concentration of sperm necessary for fertility is higher than in normal males. The minimal concentration of normal sperm necessary for fertility in normal women is probably much lower than 20 million/ml. It is not known whether increasing the concentration of normal or abnormal spermatozoa above the so-called minimum can improve the fertility of subfertile women. Adequate amounts of seminal fluid are desirable for neutralizing the acidity of the vaginal fluid. A period of sexual rest is recommended for the treatment of infertility when the volume of the ejaculate is below normal range.

7. SURVIVAL OF SPERMATOZOA

It has been estimated that the average survival of motile human spermatozoa in the human female reproductive tract is 2.5 h in the vagina, 48 h in the cervix, 24 h in the uterus, and 48 h in the oviduct (Figure 6).

Once ejaculation has occurred spermatozoa have only a finite life span. Certain components of the seminal plasma stimulate sperm motility whereas others inhibit motility. Postcoital survival of spermatozoa in the female reproductive tract is an important factor in human fertility (Sobrero and MacLeod 1962). Much information is known about the duration of spermatozoal motility, but little is known about the duration of their fertilizing capacity, which is lost long before motility. There is a relationship between the pH of the intravaginal seminal pool and the motility of spermatozoa. Contamination with mucus at times alters the pH of the posterior fornix of the vagina and prolongs the survival of ejaculated sperm. When the pH of the pool is 6 or higher, appreciable numbers of motile spermatozoa are encountered in the vagina (Kremer 1968).

Wallace-Haagens et al. (1975) studied sperm survival in terms of numbers, motility, viability, and metabolic activity in vaginal washings obtained daily from healthy, fertile, married women during one complete menstrual cycle. The num-

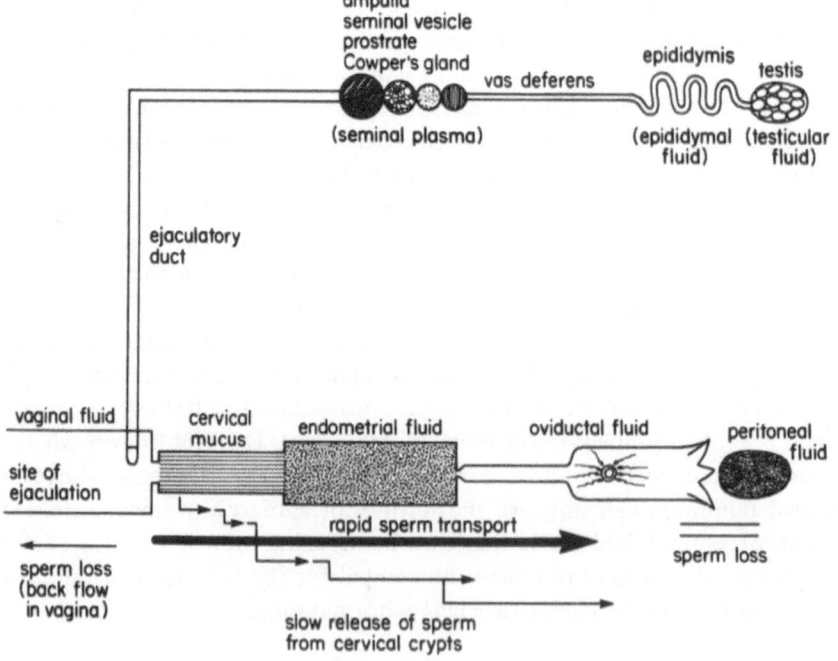

Figure 6. Diagrammatic illustration of sperm transport in the male and female reproductive tracts.

bers of sperm were never large compared to the number of sperm in a single ejaculate. Forty-eight hours after intercourse, only 6% of the specimens showed any evidence of sperm. Motile sperm were observed in only six of 94 postcoital specimens examined within 12 hours of intercourse. The small numbers of spermatozoa in the vagina after intercourse quickly become inactivated.

Sperm motility persists in the human cervix longer than in other regions of the genital tract. Motile spermatozoa, commonly observed in cervical mucus 24 h following intercourse, were found in the cervical mucus for as long as 5 days after insemination (Nicholson 1965). Motile spermatozoa were recovered from the oviduct 60 to 80 h after intercourse (Ahlgren 1969). It is unlikely that spermatozoa maintain their fertilizability for that long.

The viability of spermatozoa in vitro is related to the glucose concentration of cervical mucins (Kellerman and Weed 1970). There is an increase in glucose concentration in the cervical mucus at the time of ovulation and a decrease in many infertile women. During the fertile period, cervical mucus contains 200 mg per 100 ml of glucose or more and unexplained cervical mucus. In postcoital tests sperm viability was low in women with a low glucose content in the cervical mucus.

When migrating in the genital tract, sperm are rapidly separated from the seminal plasma and are resuspended in the female genital fluid. In the oviduct, spermatozoa are highly diluted. Since only a few spermatozoa appear in the oviduct, their survival time is difficult to estimate, and if they remain motile, they then migrate into the peritoneal cavity. Oxygen uptake of rabbit spermatozoa was higher in oviductal fluid than in saline diluent plus glucose.

During transport to the site of fertilization, spermatozoa are significantly diluted with luminal secretions from the female reproductive tract and are susceptible to changes in the pH of luminal fluids. Acidity or excessive alkalinity (above pH 8.5) of the mucus immobilizes spermatozoa, whereas moderately alkaline mucus enhances their motility. The pH range of normal midcycle cervical mucus (pH 7 to 8.5) is optimum for sperm migration and survival. Follicular, oviductal, peritoneal, and amniotic fluids have been noted to increase the activity and speed of propulsion of spermatozoa.

Glycolytic and metabolic enzymes in the sperm tail and respiratory enzymes in the mitochondria are required for the biochemical reactions of the Embden-Meyerhof pathway, the tricarboxylic acid cycle, fatty acid oxidation, and the electron transport system.

The cervical mucus secreted at the time of ovulation provides an environment suited to the maintenance of metabolic activity of spermatozoa. This mucus undergoes biochemical changes, such as a decrease in albumin, alkaline phosphatase, peptidase, antitrypsin, esterase, and sialic acid, as well as an increase in mucins and NaCl. The main components rendering mucus suitable as a 'culture medium' for sperm have not yet been identified, although hexosamines and carbohydrates existing in either a free or polysaccharide form may contribute to sperm longevity in the cervix.

Transport of spermatozoa into the uterus may influence capacitation in that the sperm are separated from an excess of the 'decapacitation factor' and from other enzyme inhibitors in the seminal plasma.

8. CONCLUDING REMARKS

The vaginal environment is hostile to sperm survival. Sperm transport through the cervix is affected by contractile activity of vagina and cervix, the properties of cervical mucus, the directional motility of sperm, and possibly orgasm. Stimulation of the female before insemination, through neurohumoral pathways, may activate rapid transport of sperm. Little is known about the factors which control sperm transport in the oviduct, for instance, about the countercurrent of oviductal fluids created by abovarian beat of cilia, peristalsis and anti-peristalsis of oviductal musculature, and contraction of mucosal folds and mesosalpinx. Several methods have been adopted to study sperm distribution in the human female reproductive tract through laparotomy or laparoscopy. Spermatozoa, aided by myometrial contraction, may reach the site of fertilization within 2-10 minutes. During their transport in the female tract spermatozoa are separated from seminal plasma and resuspended in endometrial and oviductal fluid; this reduces survival time of sperm. Sperm transport is affected by endocrine, hereditary, immunological and psychological factors. Massive numbers of spermatozoa enter the endometrial glands or undergo phagocytosis by the leukocytes. A continual sperm loss occurs into the vagina and peritoneal cavity.

REFERENCES

Ahlgren A: Number of spermatozoa in the ampulla of the human fallopian tube. *World Cong Fertil Steril* Tokyo, 1971.

Ahlgren M: *Migration of spermatozoa to the fallopian tubes and the abdominal cavity in women including some immunological aspects,* Lund: Student Literatur, 1969.

Bakker RD, Degen AA: Transport of live and dead boar spermatozoa within the reproductive tract of gilts. *J Reprod Fertil* 28:369-377, 1978.

Boer CH de: Transport of particulate matter through the human female genital tract. *J Reprod Fertil* 28:295-297, 1972.

Davajan V, Nakamura RM, Kharma K: Spermatozoan transport in cervical mucus. *Obstet Gynecol Survey* 25:1-43, 1970.

Eliasson R, Posse N: The effect of prostaglandin on the nonpregnant human uterus in vivo. *Acta Obstet Gynecol Scand* 39:112-126, 1960.

Frenkel DA: Sperm migration and survival in the endometrial cavity. *Int J Fertil* 6:285, 1961.

Hafez ESE: Scanning electron microscopy of the female reproductive tract. *J Reprod Med* 9:119-122, 1972.

Hafez ESE: The comparative anatomy of the mammalian cervix. In: *The biology of the cervix*, Blandau RJ, Moghissi KS (eds), Chicago, University of Chicago Press, 1973a.

Hafez ESE: Gamete transport. In: *Human reproduction: conception and contraception*, Hafez ESE, Evans TN (eds), New York, Harper and Row, 1973b, p 85-118.

Hafez ESE: Sperm transport. In *Progress in infertility*, Behrman, SJ, Kistner RW (eds), Boston, Little, Brown, 1975.

Hafez ESE: Transport and survival of spermatozoa in the female reproductive tract. In: *Human semen and fertility regulation in men*, Hafez ESE (ed), St. Louis, Mosby, 1976.

Hafez ESE, Thibault C (eds): *The biology of spermatozoa: maturation, transport and fertilizing ability*, Basel, Karger, 1975.

Jaszczak S, Hafez ESE: Hormonal and generative functions of transplanted ovaries in the rabbit and monkey. *Am J Obstet Gynecol* 115-112, 1973.

Kellerman AS, Weed JC: Sperm Motility and survival in relation to glucose concentration: an in vitro study. *Fertil Steril* 21:802-805, 1970.

Kremer J: *Sperm penetration in cervical mucus*, Fertility investigation thesis 24, Groningen, Van Denderen, 1968.

Masters WH, Johnson VE: *Human sexual response*, Boston, Little, Brown, 1966.

Moghissi KS: Sperm transport in the human cervix. In: *Biology of the cervix* Blandau RJ, Moghissi KS (eds), Springfield (Ill), Thomas, 1973.

Nicholson R: Vitality of spermatozoa in the endocervical canal. *Fertil Steril* 16:758-764, 1965.

Odeblad E: The physics of the cervical mucus. *Acta Obstet Gynecol Scand* 38 (suppl 1): 44, 1959.

Odeblad E: Micro-NMR in high permanent magnetic fields. *Acta Obstet Gynecol Scand* 45 (suppl 2): 12, 1966.

Odeblad, E.: The functional structure of human cervical mucus. *Acta Obstet Gynecol Scand* 47 (suppl 1): 57, 1968.

Schumacher GFB: Biochemistry of cervical mucus. *Fertil Steril* 21:697-705, 1970.

Schumacher GFB, Pearl MJ: Alpha$_1$ antitrypsin in cervical mucus. *Fertil Steril* 19:91-99, 1968.

Sobrero AJ: Sperm migration in the human female. In: *Fertility and sterility; proceedings of the fifth world congress*, Westin B, Wiqvist N (eds), Amsterdam, Excerpta Medica, 1967.

Sobrero AJ, MacLeod J: The immediate post-coital test. *Fertil Steril* 13:184-189, 1962.

Tredway DR, Settlage DSF, Nakamura RM, Motoshima M, Umezaki CU, Mishell DR: Significance of timing for the postcoital evaluation of cervical mucus. *Am J Obstet Gynecol* 121:387-393, 1975.

Wallace-Haagens MJ, Duffy Fr BJ, Holtrop JR: Recovery of spermatozoa from human vaginal washings. *Fertil Steril* 26:175-179, 1975.

3. IN VITRO SPERM PENETRATION IN CERVICAL MUCUS AND AIH

J. KREMER

An in vitro sperm penetration test with the semen of the husband and the cervical mucus of the wife is useful in order to know whether artificial insemination with the husband's semen has a reasonable chance of achieving a pregnancy and to know which type of insemination (intravaginal, intracervical or intrauterine) is to be preferred.

The earliest in vitro sperm penetration test, which is still used in many clinics because of its simplicity, is described by Miller and Kurzrok (1932). The most convenient method of performance of this test is, in my experience, as follows. The cervical mucus is collected during the preovulatory phase of the menstrual cycle. The uterine cervix is put in position by means of a vaginal speculum. The external os is cleaned with a piece of dry gauze, which is kept in a dressing forceps. A tuberculine syringe is introduced into the cervical canal in such a way that the conus is inside the canal while the end of the syringe is lightly pressed against the cervix. As much mucus as possible is aspirated into the syringe. Before the syringe is drawn back the plunger must be released in order to break the vacuum, otherwise air bubbles, vaginal contents and sometimes blood will be mixed with the cervical mucus. Evaporation of the mucus and contamination with micro-organisms is prevented by putting a thin needle, provided with a cap, on the syringe. In this way the material can be stored in the refrigerator for 48 hours without alteration of the test results.

The semen is obtained by masturbation, after a period of continence of 3-5 days, since a shorter time makes it difficult for some men to induce the ejaculation reflex. Hands and penis are washed beforehand and dried afterwards, because water and soap have an unfavourable influence on sperm motility. Micturition should not have taken place less than one hour before the masturbation in order to prevent urine, which would otherwise still be present in the urethra during the ejaculation, being mixed with the semen.

The semen is collected in a small, dry, cylindrical bottle of glass or plastic. The bottle must be brought to about body temperature before the ejaculation, since a sudden drop in temperature can cause an irreversible shock for spermatozoa. The diameter of the bottle must be between 3 and 4 cm. If it is not possible to collect the semen in the building where the test will be performed, then special arrangements must be taken to prevent damage of the spermatozoa. The semen must be delivered to the laboratory within one hour of the ejaculation. During transport the semen must be kept cool in order to avoid loss of energy. To avoid too much contact between spermatozoa and air, which impairs spermatozoal motility, violent shaking must be prevented during the transport. The screwtop of the bottle must be constructed in such a way that spillage of semen during the transport is impossible.

The microscopic slide on which the Miller-Kurzrok test is performed must be clean, dry and free of chemicals. A drop of the cervical mucus in the syringe is pushed through the thin needle onto the microscopic slide. The pressure necessary to push the mucus through the needle gives an impression of the viscosity of the cervical mucus. Normal preovulatory cervical mucus needs only light pressure on the syringe plunger to pass through the thin needle. A coverslip is put on the cervical mucus; by light pressure on this the mucus is spread as a thin film under the coverglass. A drop of semen, placed at the edge of the coverglass, flows under it by means of capillary force and makes a boundary line with the cervical mucus. The slide is put under the microscope and the boundary line between mucus and semen is brought in the microscopic viewing field.

When normal semen and normal preovulatory cervical mucus are used, sperm penetration, occurring in groups of spermatozoa, starts after a short time (Miller and Kurzrok 1932). Each group forms a kind of spearhead, for which the term *phalanx* was used. These phalanxes penetrate more and more deeply into the cervical mucus. The formation of phalanxes was considered by Miller and Kurzrok as being the result of spermatozoal activity, but it was shown by Perloff and Steinberger (1963) that phalanx formation also occurs in cases of azoo-spermia. They were able to render this visible by the addition of a dye (India ink) to a spermatozoa-free ejaculate and by performing a Miller-Kurzrok test with this material. From this it appeared that phalanx formation is a physical phenomenon which is due to the filling-up of 'inlets' in the cervical mucus. Although the Miller-Kurzrok test can give a good impression regarding the penetration capacity of spermatozoa and the penetrability of the cervical mucus, the results of this test cannot be used to obtain exact information about the migration distance, the penetration density or the duration of motility of the spermatozoa. These data can be obtained by using a *capillary method* instead of a coverslip method. Lamar et al. (1940) utilized glass capillaries with an internal diameter of 0.1-0.4 mm. A small quantity of cervical mucus was sucked into the capillary tube, followed by an air bubble and then by a small quantity of fresh semen. The glass capillary hence contained a column of cervical mucus and a column of semen, separated by a small air bubble, which was required to prevent mixing of mucus and semen and marked a clearly visible boundary between the two liquids. Provided the air bubble was small enough, sufficient mucus was left adhering to the wall of the glass capillary to ensure a contact zone between cervical mucus and semen. By placing the capillary tube under a microscope, the penetration of the spermatozoa into the cervical mucus could easily be observed. In a modified technique (Schwartz and Zinsser 1954, 1955), semen and cervical mucus were no longer separated from each other by an air bubble. The glass capillary, which was closed at both ends, was kept at a temperature of 37° C under a microscope, the viewing stage being set in a vertical position. The disadvantage of these capillary methods, however, is the difficulty of sucking semen and cervical mucus one after the other into the same capillary tube, because of the difference in viscosity between the two liquids.

Botella-Llusia (1956) described the results obtained by a Spanish-Mexican group of workers with the in vitro spermatozoal penetration test. The most important difference from the capillary methods already described was that semen and cervical mucus (or another medium) were each placed in a separate reservoir. The test was performed as follows. A small quantity of semen was pipetted into the cavity of a hollow ground-glass slide. A glass capillary tube, filled with cervical mucus or Ringer's solution was sealed at one end with paraffin and the other end was placed in the drop of semen on the glass slide, in a horizontal or vertical position. The whole system was incubated at 37° C for 30 minutes. The capillary was then examined microscopically to see how far the spermatozoa had penetrated into the medium in question.

In 1965 an apparatus with which one could determine the *migration distance, the penetration density, the migration reduction, and the duration of progressive movements* of spermatozoa in cervical mucus or in another medium was developed (Kremer 1965). The construction of this apparatus, called a sperm penetration meter, was very simple. A small test tube with a length of approximately 7 cm and an external diameter of approximately 8 mm (a so-called serum tube, often used for blood group investigation) was sawn lengthwise for a distance of 1 cm from the bottom by means of a rotating glass-saw. Care was taken that the saw did not pass exactly through the middle of the tube, because then two identical halves were produced, which however, were both too small for the envisaged use (part of the glass, equivalent to the thickness of the glass saw, is removed). The test tube was sawn in such a way that one of the side surfaces of the glass-saw passed exactly through the middle of the tube. The tube was then sawn through at right angles to the longitudinal sawcut at a distance of 1 cm from the bottom. In this way two unequal bottom pieces, each with a length of 1 cm, were obtained. The bigger one was fixed into a calibrated glass slide with glass glue, slightly above the midpoint of one of the short sides. The open section of the little reservoir formed in this way faced the other short side and ran parallel to it. A glass rod with a length of 2 cm and a diameter of 1 mm was glued to the glass slide at a distance of 1 cm from, and parallel to, the open section of the small glass reservoir.

This sperm penetration meter proved in our laboratory to be a suitable apparatus to perform in vitro spermatozoal penetration tests. The test was used

for research work and for routine fertility investigations. The results were published by Kremer (1968). The sperm penetration meter underwent some modifications during the period 1968-1975, the most important being the replacement
of the circular capillary tubes by square ones (Kremer and Kroeks 1974) and
later by flat rectangular ones. These tubes are produced in different sizes by Vitro
Dynamics Inc., 114 Beach Street, Rockaway, New Jersey 07866, US. The advantage of a rectangular tube over a circular one is the prevention of the
distortion of sperm in the microscopic picture caused by a curved glass wall. The
present model of the sperm penetration meter (J. de Groot, Kastanjelaan 1,
Harmelen, The Netherlands: $ US 5.00) is provided with three semen reservoirs.
It has a level reduction of about 1 cm in length just in front of the reservoirs
(Figure 1); this construction prevents the semen from flowing out of the semen
reservoir into the thin cleft between the slide and the capillary tube by means of
capillary force.

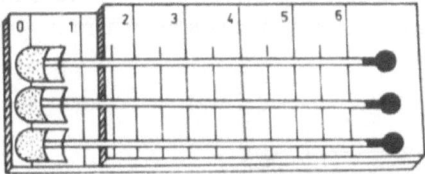

Figure 1. Sperm penetration meter with 3 semen reservoirs. The apparatus has the size of a slide and
can be examined under a microscope; the semen reservoirs are small enough to retain the contents if
the apparatus is in a horizontal position. The glass capillaries can be filled with cervical mucus or
other penetration fluids.

Migration distance, penetration density and migration reduction are read and
registered after two hours incubation at 37° C. Duration of progressive movements is read and registered after 2, 6, 24 and 48 hours of incubation. I will
describe very briefly now how these four aspects of 'cervical mucus-sperm
interaction' are examined and embodied.

Migration distance is the distance from the beginning of the capillary tube to
the foremost spermatozoa. This distance is expressed in distance groups:

    0 cm migration: group 0;
    <1 cm migration: group 1;
    1–2 cm migration: group 2;
    2–3 cm migration: group 3;
    3–4 cm migration: group 4;
    >4 cm migration: group 5.

Penetration density is expressed as the mean of the estimated number of
spermatozoa in 5 low-power fields (ocular 10, object lens 10). The area in the

capillary tube where density appears to be highest is used for the estimation, this being usually the first part of the capillary tube but this is not always the case. Penetration is expressed in density classes:

           0 spermatozoa: class 0;
    0–   5 spermatozoa: class 1;
    6– 10 spermatozoa: class 2;
   11– 20 spermatozoa: class 3;
   21– 50 spermatozoa: class 4;
   51–100 spermatozoa: class 5;
   > 100 spermatozoa: class 6.

   Migration reduction indicates the decrease of penetration between 1 cm and 4.5 cm from the semen reservoir. This decrease is expressed in *reduction points*. The number of reduction points is the difference between the density class at 1 cm and at 4.5 cm, so there is no reduction if the density at 4.5 cm is the same or higher than at 1 cm (Figure 2). Duration of progressive movements is the time of the reading at which progressive movements somewhere in the capillary tube are noticed for the last time.

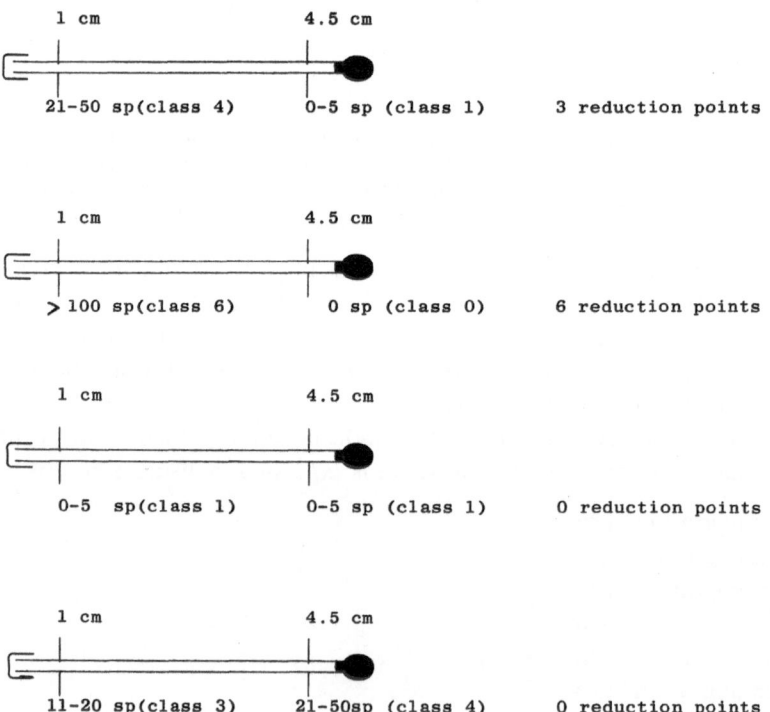

Figure 2. Four examples of the assessment of migration reduction.

The four different data from the sperm penetration meter test are combined in order to assess the end result of the test. This classification can be *negative*, *poor*, *fair* or *good*. Table 1 shows a convenient quick classification. The result of the in vitro sperm penetration test can play a role in the decision to perform AIH and also in the choice of the insemination technique. It seems reasonable to perform intracervical inseminations in infertile couples with a poor postcoital test but a good in vitro sperm penetration test. Intrauterine inseminations look to be the method of choice in infertile couples with normospermia, a poor postcoital test (PCT) and also a poor in vitro sperm penetration test. Table 2, however, indicates that this presupposition is not true. In 13 infertile couples with a poor PCT and a poor in vitro penetration test, we achieved only one pregnancy by intrauterine inseminations. On the other hand, in a group of 9 infertile couples with a poor postcoital test but a fair or good in vitro sperm penetration test we could achieve 6 pregnancies by intrauterine inseminations. In 12 couples with a good result of the PCT and also a good result of the in vitro sperm penetration test, but an unexplained infertility of more than 5 years, 5 pregnancies were achieved by

Table 1. Classification of the result of the sperm penetration meter test.

Migration distance (groups)	Penetration density (classes)	Migration reduction (points)	Duration of progression (hours)	Classification
0	—	—		Negative
1, 2, 3	or 0, 1, 2	or 4, 5, 6	or <6	Poor
All combinations that cannot be classified as negative poor or good				Fair
4, 5	and 5, 6	and 0, 1, 2	and >24	Good

Table 2. Results of intrauterine inseminations in different groups of infertile couples.

Number of couples	Semen evaluation	Result of PCT	Result of in vitro penetration test	Number of preg- nancies	Remarks
13	normospermia	poor	poor	1	
9	normospermia	poor	fair/good	6	
12	normospermia	fair/good	fair/good	5	
6	subfertile	poor	fair (1×)	1	
			poor (5×)	0	
20	normospermia	poor	poor	4	sperm antibodies in 15 men and 5 women

intrauterine inseminations. In 6 couples with subfertile semen the only pregnancy was achieved in a couple with a fair result of the in vitro sperm penetration
test.

So a poor in vitro sperm penetration test in couples with normospermia seems,
surprisingly enough, not to be a good reason for intrauterine insemination,
whereas a good result of the in vitro sperm penetration test promises a better
chance of success. This postulate is probably also valid for infertile couples where
a poor result of the in vitro sperm penetration test is due to the presence of sperm
antibodies in the semen or in the cervical mucus. In 20 such couples, the last
group in the table, only 4 pregnancies were obtained by intrauterine inseminations. In one of these couples the antibodies were found in the cervical mucus and
in 3 couples in the semen. The four couples for whom a pregnancy was achieved
had been infertile for a period of 3-8 years. In each of these four couples the
postcoital test and the in vitro sperm penetration test was performed at least four
times and in none of the tests was progressively moving sperm found, although
semen qualities and cervical mucus qualities were quite normal.

SUMMARY

The results of an in vitro sperm penetration test with the sperm penetration
meter is composed of measurements of migration distance, penetration density,
migration reduction and duration of progressive movements. The combination
of these four parameters results in the following classification: *negative, poor, fair*
or *good*. The results of intrauterine insemination proved to be better in cases with
a fair or good result of the in vitro sperm penetration test than in cases with a
poor or negative result. This is an indication that the storage function of cervical
mucus for spermatozoa is not only important after coitus, intravaginal and
intracervical insemination, but also after intrauterine insemination.

REFERENCES

Botella-Llusia J: Measurement of linear progression of the human spermatozoon as an index of male
    fertility. *Int J Fertil* 1:113, 1956.
Kremer J: A simple sperm penetration test. *Int J Fertil* 10:209, 1965.
Kremer J: The in vitro spermatozoal penetration test in fertility investigations. Thesis, Groningen,
    The Netherlands, 1968.
Kremer J, Kroeks MVAM: Modifications of the in vitro spermatozoal penetration test by means of
    the sperm penetration meter. *Acta Eur Fert* 6:377-380, 1074.
Lamar JK, Shettles LB, Delfs E: Cyclic penetrability of human cervical mucus to spermatozoa in
    vitro. *Am J Physiol* 129:234, 1940.
Miller EG, Kurzrok R: Biochemical studies of human semen III: factors affecting migration of sperm
    through the cervix. *Am J Obstet Gynecol* 24:19, 1932.

Perloff WH, Steinberger E: In vivo survival of spermatozoa in cervical mucus. *Am J Obstet Gynecol* 88:439, 1963.
Schwartz R, Zinsser H: Sperm motility: a simple method for analysis. *Am J Med* 17:124, 1954.
Schwartz R, Zinsser H: Some factors modifying sperm progression. *Fertil Steril* 6:450, 1955.

4. PREDICTION AND DETECTION OF OVULATION: PHYSIOLOGICAL AND CLINICAL PARAMETERS

E.S.E. HAFEZ

There are 400,000 ova in a female at puberty, but there will only be 400 eggs ever used potentially for ovulation and conception (Hafez 1978b, 1980). Under the influence of FSH and LH secretion, the ovarian follicle grows and migrates to the surface of the ovary, whereupon meiosis is resumed, reducing the number of chromosomes in the nucleus from 46 to 23. The process is completed within 48 hours of ovulation. A surge of pituitary LH causes rupture of the follicle and release of the ovum from the ovary. Ovulation occurs under the influence of several physioanatomical, neural and endocrine mechanisms (Coutinho and Maia 1972; Diaz-Infante et al. 1974; Jaszczak and Hafez 1973; Neilson et al. 1970; O'Shea and Phillips 1974; Owman et al. 1975; Walles et al. 1975a, 1975b).

Ovulation detection is an important gynecological examination for artificial insemination. The presence of a mature ovarian follicle is generally not detectable by rectovaginal examination. A sudden and brief pain during midcycle in one fossa iliaca may be a sign of ovulation.

The most accurate method of detecting ovulation is the incidence of pregnancy or direct visualization of the ovarian surface with subsequent recovery of an egg from the female reproductive tract. Several indirect clinical and laboratory techniques have been used to predict and/or detect ovulation (Figure 1): biophysical and biochemical characteristics in cervical mucus (ferning, spinnbarkeit), preovulatory endocrine profile (midcycle LH surge, urinary estrogen or LH, pregnandiol excretion), basal body temperature shift (BBT), appearance of secretory endometrium, ultrasonic examination of the ovaries, and laparoscopy (Hafez 1978a, 1978b). However, none of these parameters singly or combined can be considered as conclusive. The laparoscopic examination of the ovary facilitates a direct visualization of the ovarian surface and inspection of the corpus luteum. Definite diagnosis of ovulation is still very difficult by indirect laboratory techniques, particularly in women with pelvic endometriosis.

1. CERVICAL MUCUS

At ovulation time, the cervical epithelium is under maximal estrogenic influence: the cervical mucus is most copious and its water content approaches 98%. A

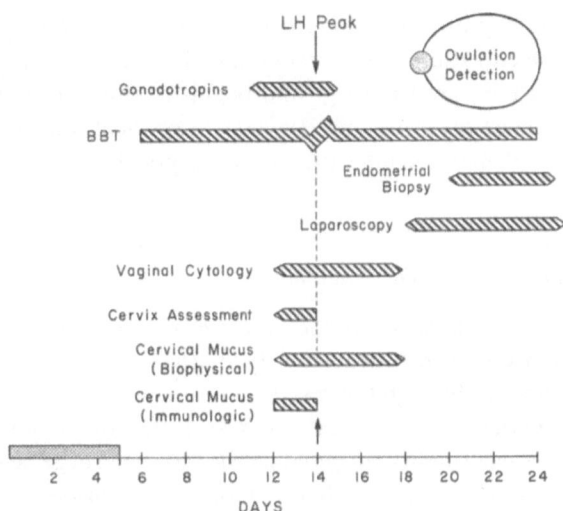

Figure 1. The various methods used for clinical detection of ovulation and the period of their applicability through the menstrual cycle.

simple technique of serial evaluation of the cervical score can be used to detect ovulation. The cervix is inspected with a vaginal speculum, and a specimen of mucus is taken with a glass pipette. A cervical score (0 to 3) is made for each of four parameters: amount of mucus, its spinnbarkeit, its ferning, and the degree of opening of the external cervical os.

Cervical mucus is made of two phases of distinct biophysical properties. The 'gel' phase, an interwoven network of glycoprotein (mucin), is made of microfibrils and macrofibrils of variable diameter. The 'sol' phase, aqueous cervical plasma, is found (a) as a fine microlayer adjacent to the epithelium of cervical crypts in which kinocilia beat, and (b) within the micellar cavities in which sperm are transported by their directional motility to the uterine lumen.

During the menstrual cycle cervical mucus undergoes several biochemical cyclical changes which are closely correlated with ovulation, e.g., concentration of water, albumins, globulins, transferrins, lactoferrins, enzymes (alkaline phosphatase and amylase), glucose, maltose, glycogen, free fatty acids, mono-, di-, and triglycerides, phospholipids, and electrolytes (Na, Ca, K, Mg, Cu, Zn, and Fe). Under the influence of midcycle estrogens, the concentrations of most of these compounds decline – with the exception of water and certain lipids, which increase (Beller and Vogler 1960; Chretein et al. 1973; Davajan et al. 1969, 1971; Elstein 1970; Elstein and MacDonald 1970; Karni et al. 1971; Kesseru 1973; Kopito et al. 1973; Moghissi 1972; Pommerenke 1946; Schmacher 1970; Viergiver and Pommerenke 1946; Weiss 1970).

The weight of cervical mucus increases gradually during the follicular phase, reaches a peak one day after the midcycle estradiol peak and decreases after ovulation. The concentration of sialic acid and the activity of a few enzymes decreases at midcycle before LH surge and begins to rise after ovulation. It is possible that self-detection of certain enzymes in cervical mucus, particularly that of alkaline phosphatase, may provide a practical method of ovulation prediction.

1.1. Viscoelastic properties of cervical mucus

The changes in the viscoelastic properties of cervical mucus are useful in ovulation detection. A decrease in viscoelasticity of the mucus is essential to the passage of spermatozoa through the cervix.

The fluidity of cervical mucus varies tenfold over the course of the menstrual cycle, with an increase in fluidity triggered by the estrogen surge beginning three to four days before LH surge associated with the fertile period.

1.2. Viscoelasticity of cervical mucus and endocrine profile

Cyclical changes in LH, FSH, progesterone, and estradiol throughout the normal menstrual cycle are evident. LH exhibits a three-day, midcycle, pre-ovulatory surge, whereas serum progesterone rises after the LH surge to peak eight days later. FSH and estradiol levels begin to rise four to five days before LH surge to peak immediately before the LH peak. The viscoelasticity of cervical mucus, which is estrogen-dependent, decreases three to four days before LH surge associated with the estrogen rise. This decrease in viscosity of the mucus is essential for sperm transport through the cervix.

After ovulation, progesterone level and viscoelasticity of the cervical mucus rise within one to two days, and penetrability of mucus to spermatozoa is inhibited.

1.3. Ovutime tackiness rheometer

This instrument is designed to identify the midcycle fertile period through changes in the biophysical characteristics of cervical mucus (Kopito and Kosasky 1978). 'Tackiness', the cohesive force which must be overcome to shear a viscoelastic fluid, is logarithmically proportional to viscosity as measured by other devices. Ovutime grid plates have precision surfaces allowing the mucus to disperse evenly in a layer of reproducible thickness. Specimens of less than 0.1 milliliter are used for the test. The tackiness rheometer functions according to the equation:

$$\text{Viscoelasticity} = \frac{\text{shear stress (dynes/sq. cm)}}{\text{shear rate (per sec)}}$$

The numerical result represents the cohesive force required to shear the mucus.

The Ovutimer (Figure 2) is a tackiness rheometer which measures the shear rate as a function of the time required to tear apart the mucus and to overcome the tensile 'yield point' of the cervical mucus over the entire range of values. The

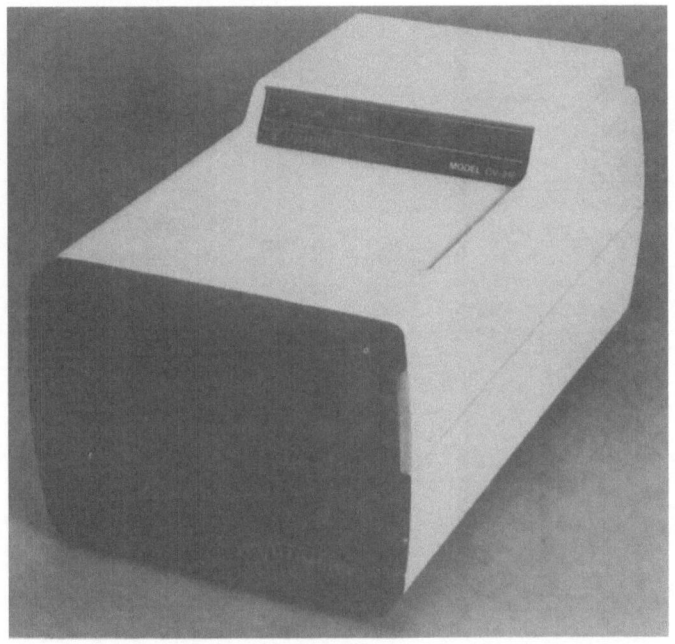

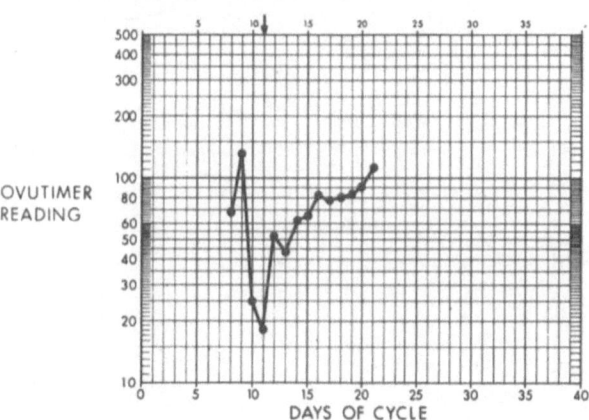

Figure 2. Ovutimer (model OV-210), a tackiness rheometer used to measure viscoelastic properties of cervical mucus to predict time of ovulation for optimal time of artificial insemination (Kopito and Kosasky 1978). Courtesy of Ovutime Inc., 1244 Boylston St., Chestnut Hill, Mass. 02167. *Bottom:* Ovutimer readings during normal ovulatory cycle.

value is displayed on the digital meter. The calibrated curve is established by the use of fluids of known viscosity.

The tackiness rheometer may be used for various purposes (see Figures 3, 4, and 5) including: (a) detection of proceeding ovulation; (b) measuring the most

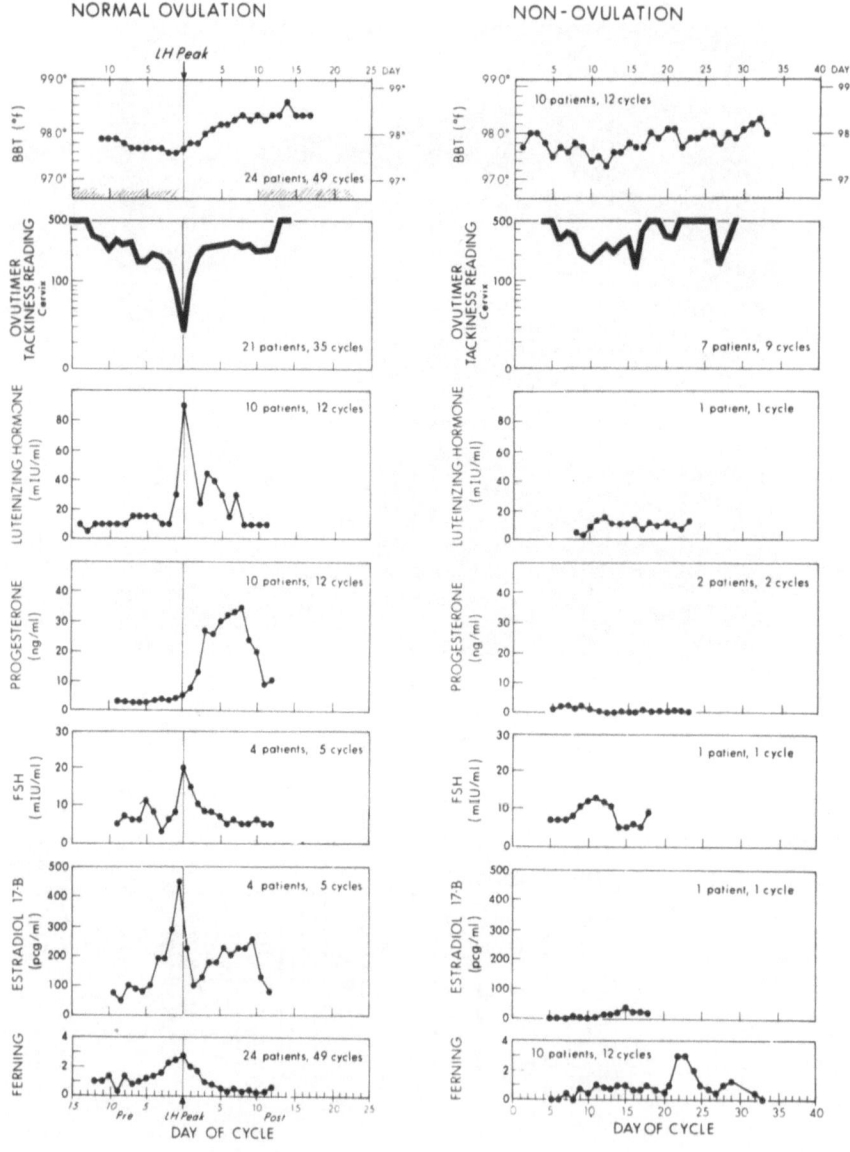

Figure 3. Endocrine profile, BBT and mucus characteristics during normal ovulation and non-ovulation (Kopito and Kosasky 1978).

fluid mucus for sperm transport; (c) recognizing anovulatory cycles; (d) detecting residual effects of steroid contraceptives; (e) identifying the optimal time for artificial insemination; (f) postcoital examinations; and (g) monitoring the effects of estrogen and other hormonal therapy (Kopito and Kosasky 1978).

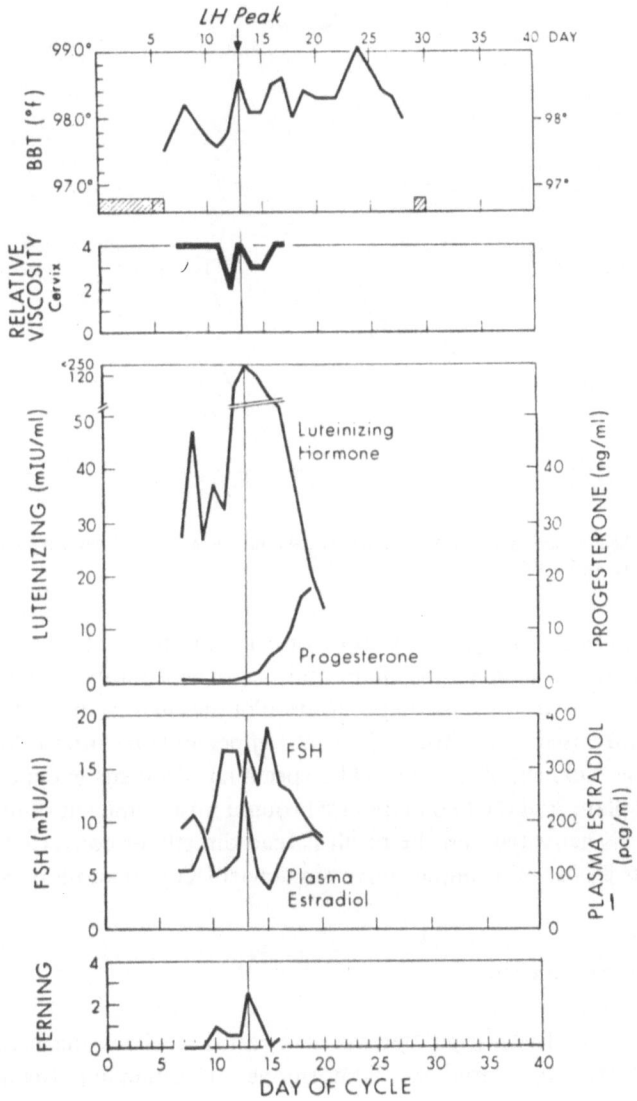

Figure 4. Endocrine profile during thick mucus syndrome (Kopito and Kosasky 1978).

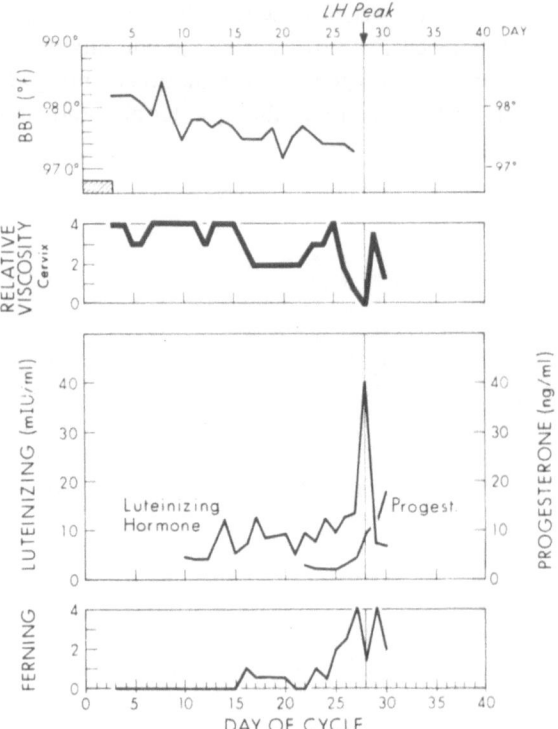

Figure 5. Cyclical variation in LH, BBT and cervical mucus characteristics during delayed ovulation (Kopito and Kosasky 1978).

1.3.1. Measuring technique. A sample of cervical mucus is removed from the external os using a warm speculum and a mucus aspirator. The specimen is forced out by extrusion, ensuring utilization of the entire sample. Two precision grid plates are used: one is inserted into the upper and one into the lower balance arms of the tackiness rheometer. The specimen of mucus is deposited on the lower grid plate, and the two plates are brought into contact at right angles. The instrument is activated and the result is read directly or converted to viscosity equivalents by use of a simple conversion chart (Kopito and Kosasky 1978).

2. ENDOCRINE PROFILE

The secretion of LH is regulated via a so-called feedback mechanism i.e., the influence exerted by ovarian steroid hormones on certain hypothalamic centers. LH and FSH are responsible for the cyclic nature of ovarian changes including ovulation and steroid production. LH is excreted in the urine and the urinary LH level can be used as a parameter of the hypophyseal secretory activities of this hormone.

2.1. Plasma steroids

Estrogens, particularly 17-β-estradiol, play an important role in triggering the LH release from the pituitary. The concentration is below 100 pg/ml in plasma during most of the follicular phase; it starts to rise a few days before the LH maximum. The values then return to a concentration which is well above the 100 pg/ml level during the luteal phase. By and large, the fluctuations of plasma estrone show a similar general pattern as that of 18-β-estradiol. There is greater variability in the maximal values for urinary estrogen, which may precede the LH peak by 1-2 days, coincide with it, or follow the peak by one day.

Significant rise of the blood levels of progesterone is not noted before the beginning of the LH discharge (Figure 6). The concentration fluctuates around 2 ng/ml plasma during the entire follicular phase. Shortly after the LH discharge starts, plasma progesterone shows a rapid rise to a plateau (about 15 ng/ml) where it remains constant during 1-3 days, after which it returns to the low levels measured during the follicular phase. Thus progesterone appears in blood only after the beginning of LH surge, but several hours before follicular rupture.

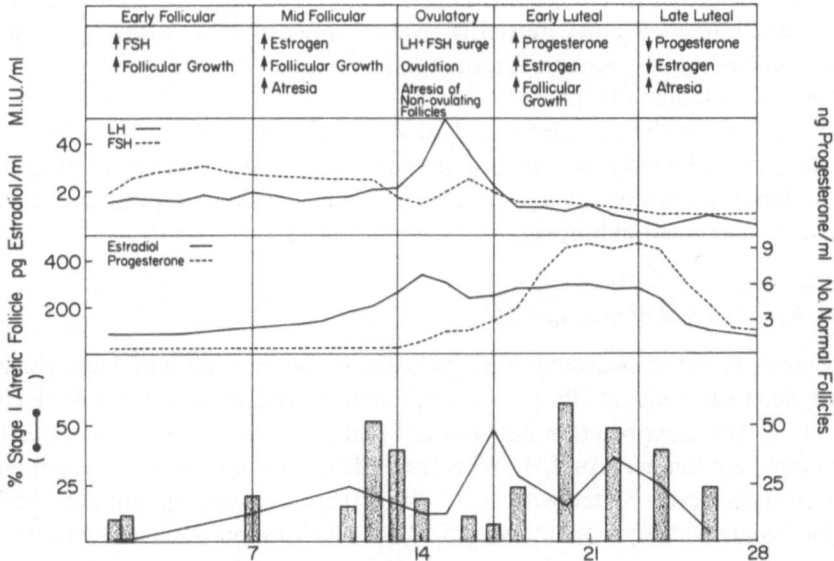

Figure 6. Endocrine profile during various stages of the menstrual cycle (From the literature and from Peluso et al. 1978).

If it is not possible to perform frequent determinations of plasma steroids, it may still be fair to conclude that a combination of low progesterone (around 2 ng/ml) and estrogen below 100 pg/ml reflects the follicular phase, whereas high estrogen in combination with low progesterone is found around the ovulation period. A combination of relatively high estrogen (above 100 pg/ml) and high levels of progesterone suggests that ovulation has already occurred.

2.2. Plasma LH

Radioimmunoassay techniques (RIA) yield specific and accurate results, however the choice and quality of antigens and antisera as well as the separation methods employed may influence the final result appreciably so that comparison of data from laboratory to laboratory becomes difficult and limited. RIA techniques which utilize sera reflect only the hormone level at a specific time period. Also there are diurnal patterns of hormone level LH excretion during a normal menstrual cycle which is characterized by an early follicular rise, and midcycle peak closely associated with ovulation. Luteal phase values are generally lower than those of the follicular phase. The midcycle LH surge normally occurs 2-48 h after the preovulatory estrogen peak and 24-72 h before the postovulatory rise in basal body temperature.

It would appear that LH peak is responsible for final ripening and release of the ovum. With luteonosticon, a local laboratory can trace a patient's LH levels and report the daily findings, including the peak, to the physician in as little as 24 hours. Luteonosticon detects LH levels as low as 9 IU/l (8 mIU/ml), and is standardized on the Second International Reference Preparation for Human Menopausal Gonadotropin.

Several methods have been used to correlate LH surge in normally menstruating females with the standard methods used for the detection of ovulation (e.g., basal temperature, cervical mucus, vaginal cytology, pregnandiol excretion, and endometrial biopsy).

2.3. Measurement of urinary LH

Urinary LH can be measured using the hemagglutination inhibition test which is designed to demonstrate the presence of human chorionic gonadotropin (HCG) in urine. The cross-reaction between LH and antiserum to HCG provides the principle for this test for LH. When anti-HCG serum (rabbit) is mixed with sheep erythrocytes coated with HCG, the erythrocytes will agglutinate. If urine which contains sufficient amounts of LH or HCG as free antigen is mixed with the antiserum, luteonosticon, commercially available, is a semi-quantitative test for luteinizing hormones in urine. It is the first immunochemical test which allows quick and accurate estimations of pituitary LH function without the need for specialized equipment and materials. The LH or HCG cross-reacts with the antibodies against HCG in the antiserum to form the antigen-antibody complex (Ag-Ab complex). When sensitized erythrocytes are added to the antigen-antibody complex, a reaction between the antibody and the antigen on the erythrocyte cannot occur since the antibodies are already bound, and agglutination is inhibited.

Because the amount of LH in unconcentrated urine is very small, the sensitivity has been amplified by permitting the immune reaction to occur in a relatively large volume of urine. An estimation of the amount of LH can easily be made by observing the shift of the end point from inhibition of agglutination to agglutination when the test is performed using dilutions of the urine specimen. Urinary LH concentration is expressed in international units (IU), immunoassay, of LH per liter of 24-h urine sample (Table 1). The sensitivity of luteonosticon has been standardized on the second International Reference Preparation for Human Menopausal Gonadotropin (2nd IRP-HMG) and will detect 8 IU (by immunoassay) of LH per liter of urine (8 mlU/ml). This sensitivity enables luteonosticon to be used in the study of normal and abnormal LH excretions. A peak value in the urinary LH excretion curve can be considered as a very important parameter, and luteonosticon can be used to detect the midcycle peak which may be absent in anovulatory cycles. If normal peaks are found it can be concluded that pituitary function is normal. In cases of amenorrhea, urine samples are collected at 3 or 4-day intervals over a two-week period. A con-

Table 1. Physiological variation in urinary LH levels as measured by immunoassay using hemagglutination inhibition techniques.

Groups	LH levels IU/24 h
Children	3 - 10
Women	
Fertile	
pre- and postovulatory	8- 50
ovulatory	50 - 200
postmenopausal	25 - 180
Men	9 - 40

stantly high LH excretion (100 lU/24 h) indicates ovarian failure, or perhaps, a pituitary tumor. If LH excretion is low or normal, additional specimens (over a 30-day period) can be examined to detect signs of cyclical activity. In patients with episodes of menstrual bleeding specimens from five days around and in cluding the fourteenth day before menstruation are tested. If no peaks are found then urine from every day of the cycle is evaluated and the baseline LH excretion estimated. Pituitary failure is characterized by constantly low or normal LH excretion and these patients are most suited for ovulation induction. The biological assays for LH and FSH are difficult to perform on urinary extracts. The reason for this is that a 24-hour specimen rarely contains enough of the hormone under investigation to inject an appropriate number of selected animals.

When exogenous gonadotropins are being administered, therapy can be monitored with luteonosticon. Daily urine specimens should be tested from the day prior to the first HCG injection for approximately eight days, or until four days after the last injection, whichever is shorter (see Figure 2). During HMG therapy, normal monitoring tests must be used to guard against the hyperstimulation syndrome prior to the HCG injections. If clomiphene therapy is being undertaken, urine specimens should be tested daily from the fourth day after cessation of therapy until a peak occurs, or for ten days, whichever is shorter. Ovulation may occur six to twelve days after cessation of therapy and is preceded by an LH peak resembling that of a normal cycle.

3. FLUCTUATIONS IN THERMOGENESIS

3.1. Basal body temperature (BBT)

BBT is used for ovulation detection to aid in both fertility and infertility problems. The cyclic thermogenesis in the female is a central phenomenon and is altered by emotion, physical activity and ovarian hormones. A rise in temperature is associated with ovulation and an LH surge.

Monophasic BBT refers to curves without a premenstrual elevated temperature but with irregular daily temperature fluctuation of 0.1. to 0.2° C. This is common in the first 20 cycles after menarche, and during premenopause as a result of ovarian dysfunction, short lifespan of corpus luteum, or deficient luteal phase. During reproductive life monophasic cycles appear singly or in clusters interspersed with biphasic BBT. Monophasic BBT is more common in short (< 17 days) and long menstrual cycles (> 60 days) than in normal cycles (25-32 days). Inadequate techniques of measurement, charting or interpretation of BBT may interfere with diagnosis of anovulatory cycles.

In the sympto-thermal method, which is more effective than BBT, fluctuations in basal body temperature are combined with cyclical changes in cervical mucus, premenstrual pain, and other related signs.

3.2. Breast temperature

There is a peak in breast temperature 2-4 days before ovulation, followed by a postovulatory increase in breast temperature. Non-breast skin temperatures do not exhibit the peak observed at the breast. Increases in breast circulation underlie the midcycle peak of breast temperature caused by preovulatory estrogen surge.

4. ENDOMETRIAL BIOPSY

Endometrial samples are obtained by simple curettage without anesthesia. Endometrial biopsies are best obtained during the ninth or tenth postovulatory day, when a well-developed secretory endometrium with typical convoluted saw-toothed glands exhibiting glandular secretion should be present. Subnuclear vacuolation, appearing within 48 hours of ovulation, does not give such reliable evidence since it may be associated with estrogen excess which may occur in the absence of ovulation.

5. VAGINAL SMEAR

Vaginal smears, collected by a standardized technique, are processed and stained using the Papanicolaou method. The vaginal epithelium undergoes remarkable changes throughout the menstrual cycle. These changes correspond to those occurring in the endometrium, but they appear slightly earlier. In the immediate postmenstrual phase the squamous cells are few in number and the smear is mainly covered by histiocytes and polymorphonuclear leucocytes. At midcycle the latter cell types disappear completely to leave a clean smear consisting almost entirely of superficial squamae, although this in itself is not diagnostic of ovulation. A few days after ovulation the vaginal smear shows mainly intermediate cells with folded edges that hang together in clumps. In the late secretory phase, just prior to menstruation, the smear becomes crowded with polymorphs.

   Evaluation of the stage of the menstrual cycle requires serial collection rather than an individual smear. Under these conditions, a sudden increase in the karyopyknotic index, KPI, which records the percentage of mature squames with pyknotic nuclei, may be the indication of the actual day of ovulation or, alternatively, a lack of change in the maturation index (which is a randomized differential count of the three).

6. CALCULATION OF PREDICTED OVULATION

Ovulation occurs 14 days before the next menstrual period. So it may be possible to give a statistical probability estimate of when the next menstrual period will occur and then subtract roughly 14 days from that. Such estimates can be determined either by calculation or from precalculated charts. The average length of several menstrual cycles is calculated.

6.1. Ovu-Guide fertility indicator

The Ovu-Guide is a small, hand-held analog calculator which is available commercially. It provides the first medically indicated method of choice to promote conception – an accurate and simple method for ovulation detection (Marshall et al. 1977).

The Ovu-Guide considers the six critical variables that are involved in fertilization and conception: menstrual cycle length, sperm viability, cervical mucus receptivity, sperm depletion, the day of ovulation, and how long the ovum lives (Figure 7). The times of longest and shortest menstrual cycles of the previous four months (or, if unknown, an appropriate approximation) together with the date of the onset of the woman's last menses. This data is automatically stored in the Ovu-Guide (Marshall et al. 1977).

Counting ahead from the specific onset date of the last menses, the Ovu-Guide identifies each of the probable days on which the next menses will begin. The Ovu-Guide fertility indicator then counts back 12-16 days from each of these projected onset days to form a mathematical distribution of all possible days on which a given woman is most likely to ovulate. Then, taking into account the following six critical variables, the Ovu-Guide indicates those days when coitus is most likely to result in conception.

Cycle length. The Ovu-Guide fertility indicator uses a woman's own individual menstrual history, which takes into account her cycle variability, to compute all the most probable expected cycle lengths and subsequent dates of the onset of menses.

Sperm viability. Even though sperm is maximally capable of fertilization for only 48 hours the frequency of AI always assures the presence of viable sperm in the female genital tract at the projected time of ovulation.

Day of ovulation. Ovulation usually precedes the onset of the menses by twelve to sixteen days.

Sperm depletion. The capacity of some men to produce sufficient sperm may be impaired by too-frequent coitus. Ejaculatory abstinence for three days prior to semen collection, and again on alternate days throughout the fertile period, is integrated into the program to ensure maximum sperm count.

Cervical mucus receptivity. Maximal receptivity of the cervical mucus to sperm occurs only during the two days preceding ovulation.

Ovum viability. Prompt fertilization of the newly-released ovum is most desirable (Marshall et al. 1977).

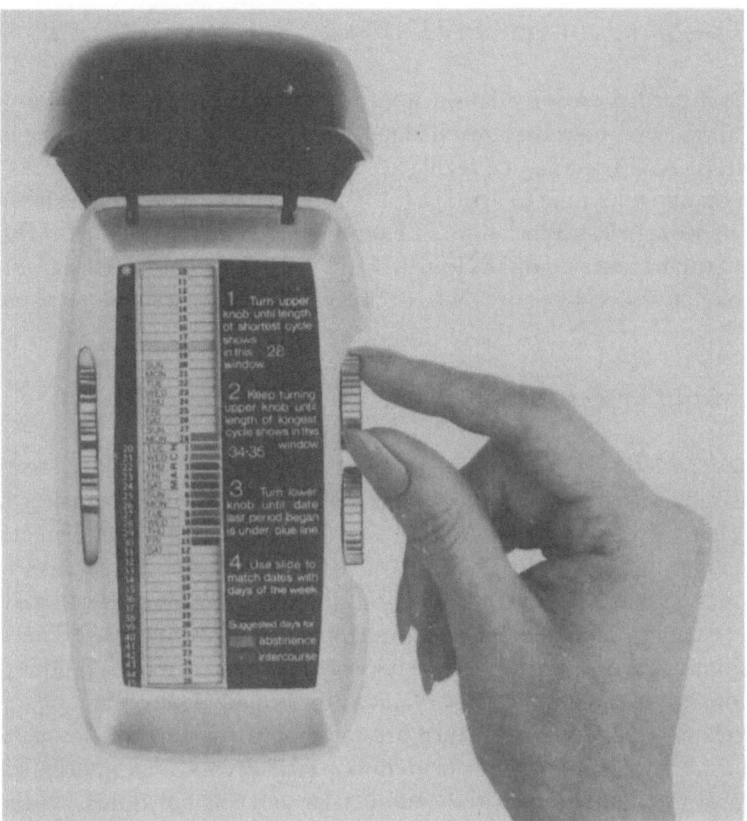

Figure 7. Ovu-Guide fertility indicator. The Ovu-Guide considers the six critical variables that are involved in enabling a woman to conceive: her cycle length, sperm viability, cervical mucus receptivity, sperm depletion, the day of ovulation, and how long the ovum lives. Consideration of all these six variables is included in the calculations of the Ovu-Guide fertility indicator (courtesy of the Reproduction Research Laboratories, Westport, Connecticut).

7. ULTRASONICS OF GRAAFIAN FOLLICLES

Ultrasonic depiction of the ovaries and the preovulatory growth of a large Graafian follicle is used to estimate the optimum time of conception especially in stimulated cycles, and to avoid a severe hyperstimulation syndrome. As the fresh corpus luteum seems to have the same ultrasonic appearance as a follicle except being somewhat smaller in diameter, reliable timing of ovulation is possible by this technique.

8. OVULATION REGULATION FOR AI

Difficulty in prediction of ovulation, improper timing of inseminations and poor insemination techniques have resulted in low pregnancy rates in patients undergoing AIH. Ovulation may be regulated and predicted within two weeks of its occurrence, allowing time to arrange for a donor and to schedule the inseminations. The woman is given 50 mg of clomiphene daily for five days. The first treatment can be initiated on the fourth, fifth, or sixth day of the menstrual cycle so that ovulation can be expected to occur on a weekday. (See also chapter 5.)

CONCLUDING REMARKS

Accurate prediction of ovulation is necessary for successful AI. Available methods require repeated AI in several cycles, however, the pregnancy rate is low. In typical cycles 4 to 5 days before ovulation the cervix is 2 cm higher in the pelvis than usual and points toward the sacrum. Two to three days before ovulation the cervical mucus undergoes remarkable biophysical and biochemical changes. The rheological parameters of cervical mucus are determined by the biophysical arrangement of the network, the diameter of backbone fibers, dimensions of secondary and tertiary microfibrils, and arrangement of aqueous intermicellar cavities, which in turn are influenced by stage of the menstrual cycle, hormonal milieu, distance from the cervical crypts, and biochemical and biophysical interactions with the endometrial and vaginal fluids. During the early follicular and luteal phases, the 'gel' phase of cervical mucus forms a three-dimensional, membranous, honeycomb-like structure that prevents sperm passage. At midcycle, these micelles appear in a prallel arrangement whereas the channels of the 'sol' phase enlarge to allow sperm migration. Cyclical changes also occur in the pattern and morphology of crystal aggregates and ferning of cervical mucus. The early follicular phase is characterized by flat, square crystals, which are rearranged during late follicular stage into parallel rows of cuboidal crystals. The concentration of sialic acid and the activity of enzymes (e.g., phosphatases, aminopeptidase, and esterase) in cervical mucus decrease at midcycle prior to LH surge and begin to rise after ovulation. Postovulatory changes include cervical mucus changes, closure of cervical os, firmness of the portio vaginalis, BBT rise, and descent of cervix to usual level.

Cyclic thermogenesis, a central phenomenon, is altered by emotion, activity, and ovarian hormones. Temperature regulation is extraordinarily complicated and a rise in temperature is associated with ovulation, a rise in LH, and increased progesterone levels. This rise in temperature may be secondary to the basic change of increased excretion of norepinephrine, which is thermogenic. Monophasic BBT (curves without a premenstrual elevated temperature but with irregular daily temperature fluctuation of 0.1 to 0.2°C) is common in postmenarcheal and premenopausal cycles, cycles with luteal deficiency, short cycles (< 17 days) and long cycles (> 60 days). Inadequate techniques of measurement, charting or interpretation of BBT may interfere with ovulation detection.

Ultrasonics have been helpful in predicting size of preovulatory follicles, but not effective in reliable detection of ovulation. Exogenous hormones have been used to release an effective LH surge, to 'program' ovulation at a 'predetermined' date of the cycle. Exogenous estrogens may improve cervical mucus receptivity to sperm, without interfering with ovulation.

REFERENCES

Beller FK, Vogler H: The consistency of human cervical mucus and its dependence on hormonal factors. In: *Flow properties of blood and other biological systems*, Copley AL, Stainsby G (eds), 1960, p 248.
Chretien FC, Gernigon C, David G, Psychoyos A: The ultrastructure of human cervical mucus under scanning electron microscopy. *Fertil Steril* 24:746, 1973.
Coutinho EM, Maia HS: Effect of gonadotropins on motility of human ovary. *Nat New Biol* 235:94, 1972.
Davajan V, Kharma K, Nakamura RM: A systematic method of diagnosing and treating the cervical factor. *J Reprod Med* III:135, 1969.
Davajan V, Nakamura RM, Mishell DR: A simplified technique for evaluation of the biophysical properties of cervical mucus. *Am J Obstet Gynecol* 109:1042, 1971.
Diaz-Infante A, Virutamasen P, Connaughton JF, Wright KH, Wallach EE: In vitro studies of human ovarian contractility. *Obstet Gynecol* 44:830, 1974.
Elstein M: The properties of cervical mucus and the influence of progestagens. *J Obst Gyn Brit Comm* 77:445, 1970.
Elstein M, MacDonald RR: The relation of cervical mucus proteins to sperm penetrability. *J Obst Gyn Brit Comm* 77:1123, 1970.
Hafez ESE: *Human reproductive physiology*, Ann Arbor (Mich), Ann Arbor Science, 1978a.
Hafez ESE: *Human ovulation: mechanisms, prediction, detection, and induction*, New York, Elsevier, 1978b.
Hafez ESE (ed): *Human reproduction: conception and contraception*. 2nd edition, Hagerstown (Md), Harper and Row, 1980.
Jaszczak S, Hafez ESE: Hormonal and generative functions of transplanted ovaries in the rabbit and monkey. *Am J Obstet Gynecol* 115:112, 1973.
Karni Z, Polishiu WZ, Adoni A, Diamant Y: Newtonian viscosity of the human cervical mucus during the menstrual cycle. *Int J Fertil* 16:185, 1971.
Kesseru E: Assessment of the rheology of cervical mucus. In: *Cervical mucus in human reproduction: WHO colloquium, Geneva, 1972*, Elstein M, Moghissi KS, Borth R (eds), Copenhagen, Scriptor, 1973, p 45.
Kopito LE, Kosaky HJ: Tackiness rheometer determination of the viscoelasticity of cervical mucus. In: *Human ovulation: mechanisms, prediction, detection induction*, Hafez ESE (ed) New York, Elsevier, 1978.
Kopito LE, Kosasky HJ, Sturgis SH, Liberman BL, Shwachman H: Water and electrolytes in human cervical mucus. *Fertil Steril* 24:4499, 1973.
Marshall JR, Langmyhr GJ, Fisher HW, Jones TL: *Coital timing and the management of infertility*, Symposium held in San Jose, California, Westport (Conn), Reproduction Research Laboratories, 1977.

Moghissi KS: The function of the cervix in fertility. *Fertil Steril* 23:295, 1972.

Neilson D, Jones GS, Woodruff JD, Goldberg B: The innervation of the ovary. *Obstet Gynecol Survey* 25:889, 1970.

O'Shea JD, Phillips RE: Contractility in vitro of ovarian follicles from sheep, and the effects of drugs. *Biol Reprod* 10:370, 1974.

Owman C, Sjoberg N-O, Svensson K-G, Walles B; Autonomic nerves mediating contractility in the human Graafian follicle. *J Reprod Fertil* 45:553, 1975.

Peluso J. Breitenecker G, Hafez ESE, In: *Atresia of ovarian follicles and ova in human ovulation: mechanisms, prediction, detection and induction*, Hafez ESE (ed.), New York, Elsevier, 1979.

Pommerenke WT: Cyclic changes in the physical and chemical properties of cervical mucus. *Am J Obstet Gynecol* 52:1023, 1946.

Schumacher GFB: Biochemistry of cervical mucus. *Fertil Steril* 21:697, 1970.

Viergiver E, Pommerenke WT: Cyclic variations in the viscosity of cervical mucus and its correlation with the amount of secretions and basal temperature. *Am J Obstet Gynecol* 51:192, 1946.

Walles B, Edvinsson L, Falck B, Owman C, Sjobert N-O, Svensson K-G: Evidence for a neuro-muscular mechanism involved in the contractility of the ovarian follicular wall: fluorescence and electron microscopy and effects of tyramine on follicle strips. *Biol Reprod* 12:239, 1975a.

Walles B, Edvinsson L, Owman C, Sjoberg, N-O, Svensson K-G: Mechanical response in the wall of ovarian follicles mediated by adrenergic receptors. *J Pharmac Exp Ther* 193:460, 1975b.

Weiss G: Effect of steroid hormones on cervical mucus. In: *Advances in steroid biochemistry and pharmacology*, Briggs HH (ed), Academic Press, 1970, p 137.

Zuspan K, Zuspan F: Basal body temperature. In: *Human ovulation: mechanisms, prediction, detection and induction*, Hafez ESE (ed), New York, Elsevier, 1978.

5. OVULATION REGULATION FOR ARTIFICIAL INSEMINATION

M.L. TAYMOR, M.J. BERGER and N.E. HAAS

1. INTRODUCTION

Careful assessment of ovulation timing is a prerequisite for artifical insemination, whether by donor (AID) or with husband's semen (AIH). In AIH, when one is dealing with semen of diminished quality, accurate timing is of special importance.

The basal body temperature chart is usually sufficient when the menstrual cycles are reasonably regular and when it is possible to carry out two inseminations per cycle (Weir and Downs 1968). For moderately irregular cycles, assessment of changes in cervical mucus provides the most practical and least expensive approach to the predetermination of ovulation (Marcus and Marcus 1963). However, when the cycles are grossly irregular hormonal endpoints become blurred, and estrogen levels, cervical mucus changes, and even LH levels (Miyata et al. 1970) lose their sharp endpoints and are thus less precise for the predetermination of ovulation. In such instances it may sometimes be more effective to induce ovulation to coincide with insemination rather than to try to predetermine the time of ovulation.

2. CLOMIPHENE CITRATE

Clomiphene citrate is one of the most widely used ovulatory-inducing agents in anovulatory women. Its effectiveness in regulating the length of cycles in women already ovulating is more open to question. When the patient is already ovulating, 50 mg of clomiphene citrate daily for 5 days, starting on the fifth day of the cycle, should induce ovulation 3-10 days after the last tablet. Three studies have been reported wherein clomiphene citrate was used in ovulatory women with irregular cycles to improve the rhythm method of contraception. In one (Boutselis et al. 1967) cycles in individual women were reported as being fairly constant, but there was a great deal of variation from patient to patient in the interval that ovulation followed clomiphene therapy. The studies of Spadoni et al. (1967) and Barzen (1968) found that in markedly irregular cycles the time interval between clomiphene therapy and onset of ovulation improved, but remained significantly irregular.

There are other drawbacks to the utilization of clomiphene for cycle regulation in conjunction with insemination therapy. The cervical mucus is often adversely affected, and this does not always respond to small doses of estrogen. Finally, a relatively high incidence of multiple pregnancies has been reported when pregnancy occurs in normal ovulating women on clomiphene (Spandoni et al. 1967).

Despite these adverse reports, in one small series a 94% pregnancy rate in 17 subjects was reported when clomiphene was used in conjunction with donor artificial insemination (Klay 1976). Another report (Tyler et al. 1975) described the use of clomiphene followed by HCG in conjunction with artificial insemination, but no results were given. Until more reports of successes as well as complications are available a guarded view should be taken as to the usefulness of clomiphene citrate in inducing ovulation in association with artificial insemination.

3. LUTEINIZING HORMONE-RELEASING HORMONE (LH-RH)

Soon after the synthesis of synthetic LH-RH it was theorized that the administration of LH-RH on a specific cycle day (e.g. 12 to 14) might induce or pinpoint ovulation (Schally et al. 1972). Preliminary reports using single injections of LH-RH to trigger ovulation were encouraging (Nakano et al. 1973), but subsequent reports (Reyes et al. 1978) as well as our own experience (Grimes et al. 1975) suggested that this approach is not universally successful. The failure of LH-RH to provoke ovulation consistently is probably due to: (1) lack of presence of a mature follicle because of the need for FSH stimulation as well as LH; (2) the short duration of the effect of LH-RH; and (3), if ovulation does occur, there is ovulation of an immature follicle.

Use of infusions of LH-RH over a four-hour period seems to bring about superior results (Gigon et al. 1973), but this is a complicated procedure for an ambulatory setting. Other approaches that might give a more prolonged LH trigger are the use of the nasal route (Nillius 1976) or of long-acting analogues (Zanartu et al. 1975), but to date there is no confirmation as to their efficacy.

4. HUMAN MENOPAUSAL GONADOTROPIN (HMG)

Human menopausal gonadotropin (HMG), followed by human chorionic gonadotropin (HCG), would seem to provide a logical, although a more inconvenient and more expensive, approach to induce ovulation. There is sufficient FSH content to provide for follicle development; there is a high concentration of endogenous estrogen to stimulate cervical mucus production; and the HCG should provide a more predictable time of ovulation.

There have been few reports as to the proper dosage of gonadotropin required – so far the treatment remains empirical. Behrman and Sawada (1966) described a case of donor insemination in a woman with irregular cycles who received 25 IU of human menopausal gonadotropin daily for 9 days and then 3,000 IU of HCG daily for 3 days. A successful pregnancy resulted. We have also previously described the use of menopausal gonadotropin in conjunction with AID in 20 patients with irregular cycles (Berger and Taymor 1971). Menopausal gonadotropin was given empirically, 150 IU daily for 5 days, starting on the eighth day of the cycle, and 5,000 IU of HCG was then administered as a single dose. Eleven of the 20 patients (55%) conceived. Since that time we have continued to use gonadotropins to induce ovulation in conjunction with insemination by both donor and homologue. Originally we used the fixed dosage approach as described above, but at a later time we utilized estrogen monitoring in conjunction with therapy in an attempt to optimize the time of HCG administration and to reduce potential complications. Results from both methods are shown in Table 1.

Table 1. Results of therapy in ovulation induction and artificial insemination using fixed dosage schedules or estrogen monitoring.

	AID	AIH
Fixed dosage		
Cases	28	11
Pregnancies	13 (40%)	2 (18%)
Twins	3	
Estrogen monitoring		
Cases	11	3
Pregnancies	5 (45%)	1 (33%)
Twins	1	

4.1. Fixed dosage

Menopausal gonadotropin (150 IU) was administered daily for five or six days starting on the seventh or eighth day of the cycle. Chorionic gonadotropin (5000-8000 IU) was then administered as a single dose the day after the last HMG injection (Figure 1). Insemination treatments were carried out two days before and on the day of the HCG injection, or on the day before and the day after the injection. Conception occurred in 13 of 28 patients (46%) treated when this method was used with donor insemination. Two of 11 patients conceived when homologous insemination was utilized.

The length of the luteal phase in 46 cycles in 19 of these patients was analyzed

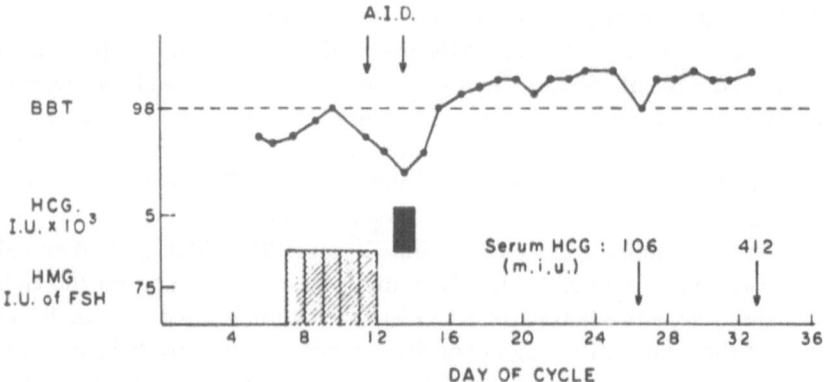

Figure 1. Flow sheet for HMG/HCG administration, for patient JB: irregular ovulator, AID, ten months of Clomid therapy.

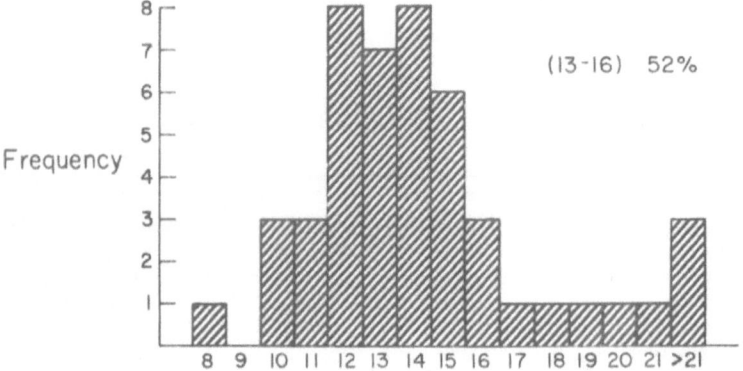

Figure 2. Frequency distribution in length of luteal phase (days) following HMG/HCG administration (46 cycles in 19 patients).

(Figure 2). Almost half the phases were less than 12 or more than 16 days in length. This suggests that the luteal phase may be abnormal in approximately half of the cycles stimulated with gonadotropin.

4.2. Estrogen monitoring

In order to optimize the time for HCG administration and possibly to improve luteal phase function, a number of patients were subjected to estrogen monitoring. HMG, 150 IU daily, was started on the third day of the cycle. On the sixth, seventh, and if necessary the eighth day of treatment, 12-hour urinary estrogen examination was measured by a rapid 6-hour method (Taymor et al.

1971). HCG was administered when the total urinary estrogen excretion reached 80 to 100 μg per 24 hours. Insemination was carried out on that day.

Five of 11 patients (45%) treated with donor insemination conceived, and one of three patients treated with homologous insemination conceived in conjunction with the gonadotropin therapy. The duration of treatment, the highest level of estrogen excretion obtained, and the length of the luteal phases are listed in Table 2. Only 4 of 11 cycles were less than 13 days in length.

Table 2. Results of treatment with HMG-HCG monitored by estrogen excretion levels.

Patient	AID/AIH	Days of HMG at 2 amp/day	Total estrogen prior to HCG	Length of luteal phase in days
SG	AID	8	101	pregnancy**
JG	AIH	9	91	pregnancy
BS	AID	5	90	11
VK	AID	9	204	12
VK	AID	8	90	pregnancy*
SS	AID	6	131	13
MM	AID	6	137	11
LM	AIH	5	97	14
RC	AIH	9	72	13
DE	AID	7	70	pregnancy
DB	AID	9	52	no ovulation
DU	AID	10	188	pregnancy
RA	AID	14	78	13
SS	AID	14	92	13

  * Blighted ovum
** Twin

3. CLOSING REMARKS

When artifical insemination is being carried out in women with irregular cycles, there is a need for approaches that will increase the chances that the insemination will be carried out close to ovulation. Methods that predict ovulation have some merit, but so far do not provide the required accuracy or consistency. For that reason, numerous attempts to force ovulation by ovulation-inducing agents have been described. These too fall short in terms of accuracy and consistency. The reports concerning the use of clomiphene citrate are few and inconclusive. On the one hand, theoretical considerations tend to lower probability of comiphene being effective, but on the other hand the one published report claims good results.

Reports concerning the use of LH-RH are even more controversial. Although the weight of evidence indicates that a single injection of LH-RH cannot trip over ovulation with significant certainty to mandate its use in conjunction with insemination, the use of more prolonged dosage regimens or of long-acting analogues does hold some promise.

The use of menopausal gonadotropin has not been widely described. Our experience indicates a modest yield in pregnancies. However, the optimum approach to therapy has yet to be described. At present there seems to be little difference in results whether or not estrogen monitoring is utilized. It can be hoped that wider interest in this mode of therapy will provoke additional reports that will dispel some of the uncertainties still present.

REFERENCES

Barzen PJ: Cycle regulation with clomiphene citrate. *Am J Obstet Gynecol* 101-1032, 1968.
Behrman SJ, Sawada Y: Heterologous and homologous inseminations with human semen frozen and stored in a liquid nitrogen refrigerator. *Fertil Steril* 17:457, 1966.
Berger MJ, Taymor ML: Combined human menopausal gonadotropin therapy and donor insemination. *Fertil Steril* 22:787, 1971.
Boutselis JG, Vorys N, Ullery JC: Control of ovulation and cycle length with clomiphene citrate. *Am J Obstet Gynecol* 97:949, 1967.
Gigon U, Stamm O, Werder H: Die Bedeutung der getimten Ovulationsinduktion mittels HCG oder synthetischen LH-RH in der Sterilitätsbehandlung. *Geburtsh Frauenheilk* 33:567, 1973.
Grimes EM, Taymor ML, Thompson IE: Induction of timed ovulation with synthetic luteinizing hormone-releasing hormone in women undergoing insemination therapy I: Effect of a single parenteral administration at mid-cycle. *Fertil Steril* 26:273, 1975.
Klay LJ: Clomiphene-regulated ovulation for donor artificial insemination. *Fertil Steril* 27:383, 1976.
Marcus LS, Marcus CC: Cervical mucus and its relation to infertility. *Obstet Gynecol Survey* 18:749, 1963.
Miyata J, Taymor ML, Levesque L, Lymeburner N: *Fertil Steril* 27:383, 1976.
Nakano R, Mizuno T, Kotsuji F, Tojo S: Triggering of ovulation after infusion of synthetic luteinizing hormone-releasing factor (LRF). *Acta Obstet Gynecol Scand* 52:269, 1973.
Nillius SJ: Therapeutic use of luteinizing hormone-releasing hormone in the human female. In: *Hypothalamus and endocrine function*, Labrie F, Meites J, Pelletier G (eds), New York, Plenum, 1976, p 93.
Reyes FI, Winter JD, Rockfort JG, Faiman C: Luteinizing hormone-releasing hormone as an ovulation trigger: problems in assessment of efficacy. *Fertil Steril* 28:1175, 1978.
Schally AV, Kastin AJ, Arimura H: The hypothalamus and reproduction. *Am J Obstet Gynecol* 114:423, 1972.
Spadoni LR, Lein JN, Herrman W: Planned ovulation: clomiphene citrate to regulate cycles in patients using the rhythm method.
Tyler Et, Friedman S, Marsh JJ: The triggering use of clomiphene with human chorionic gonadotropin and luteinizing hormone-releasing hormone in producing ovulation close to artificial insemination: abstract *Fertil Steril* 26:213, 1975.
Weir W, Downs T: The optimum time for conception. *Fertil Steril* 19:64, 1968.

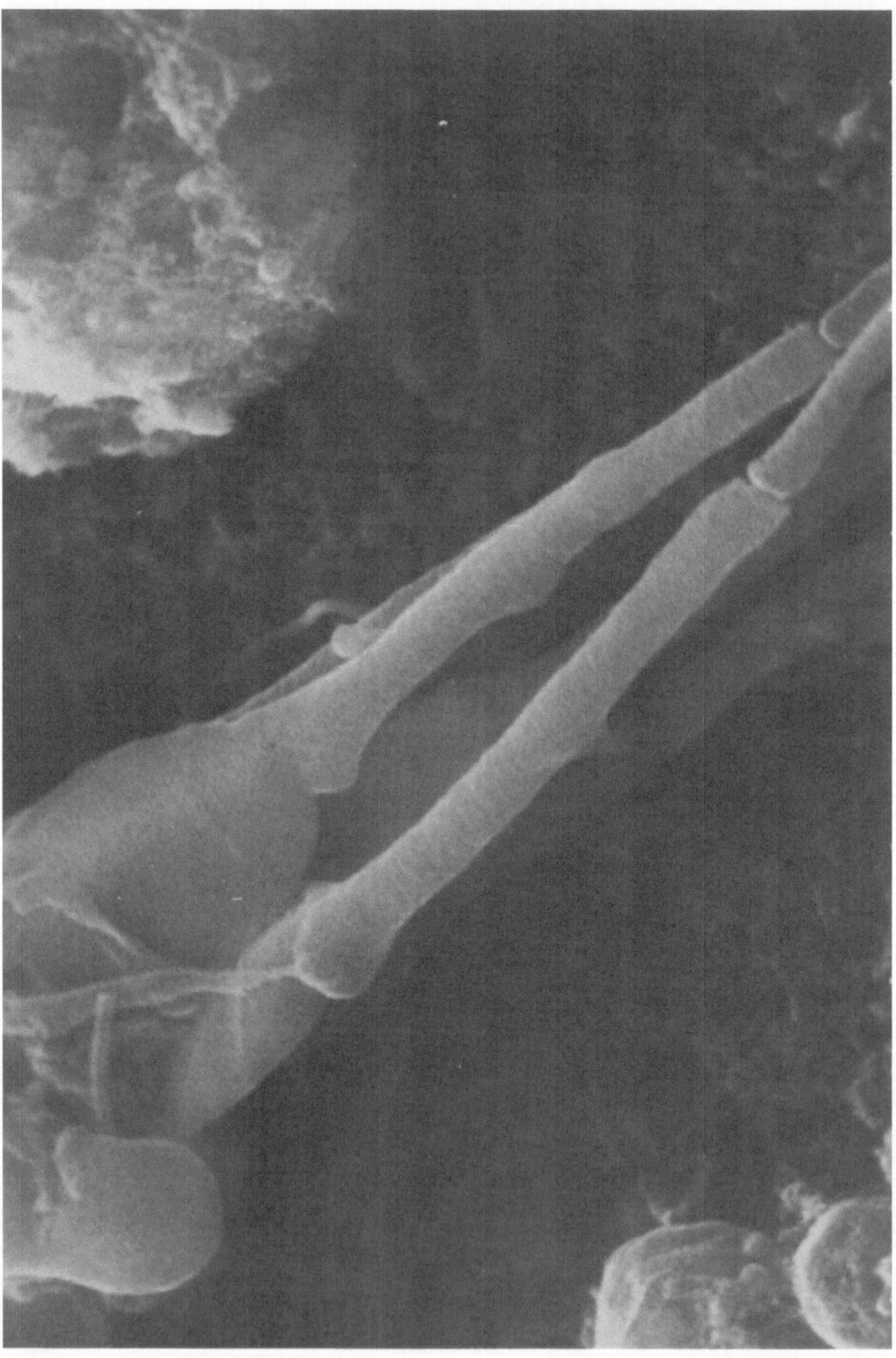

II. IN VITRO TREATMENT OF SEMEN

6. GLASS WOOL FILTRATION OF HUMAN SEMEN

J.D. PAULSON, F. COMHAIRE and J.C. EMPERAIRE

Various modes of treatment aimed at improvement of sperm production and the quality of the ejaculate of the subfertile male may be rewarding. In vivo treatment of these individuals, however, has not yielded good pregnancy rates, as often treating the cause of such problems is difficult as the etiology is unknown, so it is theoretically easier attempting to improve the specimen once ejaculated. The addition of pharmacological agents to the ejaculate yields better in vitro specimens, but the effect of insemination on pregnancy rates is still being explored. A glass wool column which increases the motility of the spermatozoa while removing dead and agglutinated spermatozoa and debris from the ejaculate has been devised and the results from its use are encouraging for specific problems.

1. SEMEN PREPARATION

1.1. Glass wool fiber

The type of glass wool used for semen filtration is important because of the different filtering properties of soda lime and borosilicate glass wool fibers. Most glass wool fiber produced is soda lime glass, but by utilizing a special process, a borosilicate glass wool of approximately .006 mm (Pyrex ®, Corning), which is stronger and more resistant to breakage into small particles, is produced. Because of its size, more soda lime glass wool fiber has to be used to achieve similar filtration for an increase in motility. Moreover impurities are removed from the Pyrex ® glass by evaporation, the temperature being raised to 300-400 C whereas glass made with soda (NaO) and lime (CaO) melts before impurities can be removed.

1.2. columns

There are three column procedures (Table 1) which have been used in laboratory and clinical work. Technique 1 (Figure 1) requires placing 40-60 mg of glass wool fiber (Pyrex ®, Corning) so that it is loosely distributed throughout but

Table 1. A summary of the various glass wool column filtration techniques' results.

	Technique 1	Technique 2a	Technique 2b	Technique 3
Initial motility	increased	increased	increased	increased
Motility after four hours	increased	decreased	increased	
Loss of motile sperm per ml	none	varied		none
Loss of total sperm per ml	33%	56%-90%		45%
Viscosity	decreased			decreased
Dead spermatozoa	removed			removed
Debris	fewer			fewer
Volume loss	0.3 ml	1.0 ml	0.2 ml	0.2 ml
Morphology	unchanged/ better	increased short tails		unchanged/ better
Clinical success			pregnancies	pregnancies
Motility after cryopreservation	better			
Cervical mucus penetration	improved			

does not extend into the tip of a disposable five-inch Pasteur pipette (Paulson and Polakoski, 1977a, 1977b). If a soda lime glass is used, it is necessary to pack the column more tightly and use more glass wool (techique 2a) to effect a filtration (Verdaquer et al. 1978). Technique 2b is an alteration of 2a derived by treating the soda lime glass wool in the packed column with 1.0 ml of a phosphate buffer solution before and after the ejaculate has been applied.

Technique 3 involves tightly packing 15-20 mg of glass wool fiber to a height of 3-5 mm into a Pasteur pipette which has been reduced in size to a length of 40-50 mm. The pipette tapers over a distance of no more than 5 mm to a 10 mm point with a diameter of 1mm (Combaire and Vermeulen 1978, unpublished). Either industrial yellow glass wool cleaned with methanol until colorless, or borosilicate glass wool may be used; they give comparable results.

1.3. Treatment of semen

A semen sample is placed on the top of the column and allowed to flow through it with no help other than the force of gravity. When utilizing a column described in techniques 1 and 2, up to 2.5 ml of semen can be placed on one column without overloading it or decreasing the effect. When using the smaller column (technique 3), only 1.0. ml should be placed on the column; several columns are used in parallel in order to filter greater volumes of ejaculate. The addition of caffeine in a final concentration of 7 mMol is known to stimulate sperm motility and to increase the lifespan of spermatozoa (Bunge 1973; Barkay et al. 1977). Caffeine has also been used by some investigators to protect the ejaculated spermatozoa during the filtration procedure and possible subsequent manipulations.

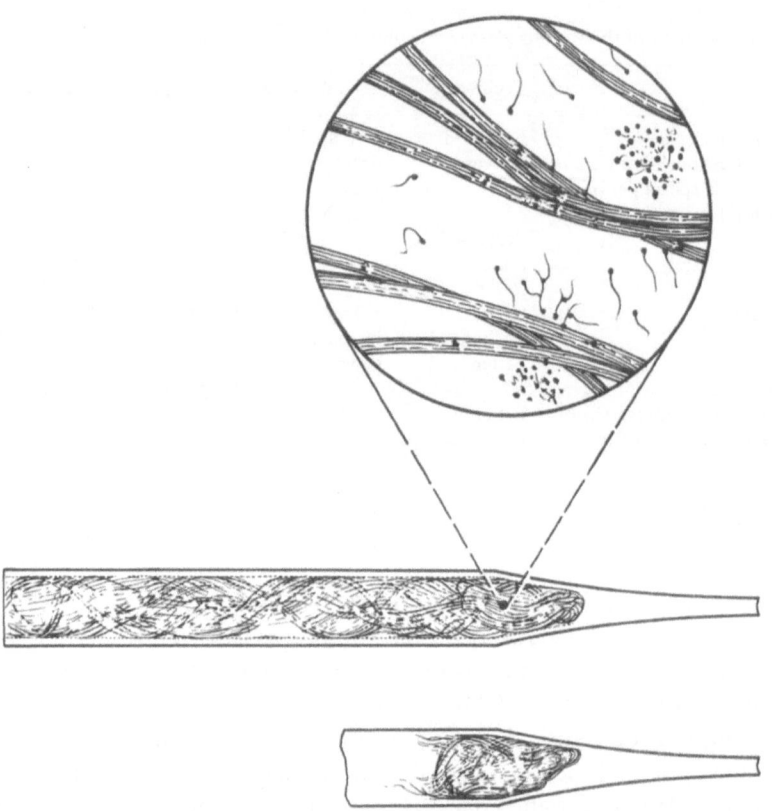

Figure 1. A representation of the glass wool column is shown. The column, a Pasteur pipette which has been shortened to approximately 4-5 cm, may be either packed tightly at the bottom (technique 3), loosely packed with a borosilicate glass (technique 1), or packed more tightly with a soda lime glass wool (technique 2). A higher magnification of the fibers shows dead spermatozoa adherent to the glass wool and debris and agglutinated spermatozoa trapped in between the fibers.

2. EFFECT ON SEMEN

2.1. Seminal components

After an ejaculate is applied to the column, it slowly traverses through the network of glass wool fibers before being collected. Microscopic examination of these fibers reveals spermatozoa adhering to the glass wool as well as debris and agglutinated spermatozoa caught within the mesh formed by these fibers (Figure 1). Use of supravital staining demonstrates that the majority of the spermatozoa stuck to the glass wool are dead (Paulson and Polakoski 1977a). Viscosity is reduced to within a normal range on viscous samples and all specimens which have flowed through the column are perfectly fluid and cleaned of mucous filaments, cellular debris and agglutinates (Paulson and Polakoski 1977a; Comhaire and Vermeulen 1978, unpublished). The material and seminal fluid left behind in the column constituted a volume loss amounting to approximately 0.2-0.3 ml utilizing either techniques 1 or 3 (Paulson and Polakoski 1977a; Comhaire and Vermeulen 1978, unpublished). When soda lime glass wool fiber is used with the first filtration technique (technique 2a) there is a loss of volume approaching 1.0 ml (Verdaquer et al. 1978). This discrepancy is most likely the result of the need to increase the amount of glass wool fiber when using soda lime glass. The loss of spermatozoa with these columns is between 56% and 90% and the total loss of motile spermatozoa is between 7% and 79% (Verdaquer et al. 1978). These losses of concentration by technique 2a utilizing soda lime fiber packed tightly are in contradistinction with the other techniques where the average loss of spermatozoa is between 33% and 45% and the concentration of motile spermatozoa per ml remains practically unchanged (Paulson and Polakoski 1977a; Comhaire and Vermeulen 1978, unpublished). By utilizing a phosphate buffer solution (technique 2b), the loss of spermatozoa is, in contrast to technique 2a, reduced to approximately 0.2 ml, leading to a higher recovery total of motile spermatozoa.

Comparison of morphology in the samples prior to and after filtration also shows differences between the various techniques. Those techniques involving borosilicate glass distributed throughout (technique 1) and glass wool tightly packed (technique 3) appear to show no alteration in the microscopic morphology; in fact, the percentage of normal spermatozoa is increased and the percentage of spermatozoa with alterations is decreased in samples after filtration (Paulson and Polakoski 1977a; Comhaire and Vermeulen 1978, unpublished). Other methods (technique 2a) show an increase in spermatozoa with short tails (Verdaquer et al. 1978), possibly due to an effect of the fiber itself, as sharp glass particles can be seen in the ejaculate after passage through the column with this type of glass wool.

2.2. Motility

When samples with decreased motility (<40% progressive) are filtered, the average percentage of progressive spermatozoa increases to greater than 65-70% (Paulson and Polakoski 1977a; Verdaquer et al. 1978; Comhaire and Vermeulen 1978, unpublished). Investigators have found that the increased motility after column filtration is maintained over a four-hour time interval (Paulson and Polakoski 1977a; Paulson et al. 1978, 1979). The use of soda lime fiber (technique 2a) appears to be deleterious to long-term survival of spermatozoa as some investigators have noted an increased motility maintained two hours after filtration, but a tremendous decrease to a level below the prefiltration motility after four hours (Verdaquer et al. 1978). This loss of motility can be counteracted by the utilization of phosphate buffer solution before and after filtration (technique 2b); the motility pattern is then similar to the other methods.

2.3. Cervical mucus penetration

In vitro cervical mucus penetration depth is improved in viscous samples after column filtration (Paulson et al. 1978, 1979). Non-viscous samples, however, show no difference in penetration depth when comparing samples before and after passage through the column. The portion of the samples which are filtered through the column and then cryopreserved and thawed demonstrates improved cervical mucus penetration in comparison to the portion of the samples that only undergoes freezing (Paulson et al. 1978a).

2.4. Cryopreservation

Semen samples undergoing cryopreservation with subsequent thawing demonstrate increased survival if filtered prior to freezing (Paulson and Polakoski 1977a; Paulson et al 1978b). The percentage of forward progressive spermatozoa and the motility percentage are significantly increased. Also, after samples with normal semen parameters have undergone cryopreservation and thawing, motility is increased by glass wool filtration.

3. CLINICAL APPLICATION

3.1. Theoretical aspects

Ejaculates with normal sperm densities, volumes and morphologies may have decreased forward motility; there are various reasons for this pathogenesis. After liquefaction of the seminal clot, a highly viscous sample may have severely diminished progressive motility as the sample's motility pattern may be reduced to moving randomly, shaking, or gyrating non-progressive movement, as the spermatozoa are trapped in a web or mesh of viscous material. Rarely, infertility can be attributed to this factor and pregnancies have resulted from various types of treatment (Amelar 1966). The marked improvement in motility of viscous samples and in those with increased agglutination should be useful for the few cases of infertility due to these causes.

In vitro cervical mucus penetration provides good correlation with fertility; there is a significant difference between the depth of penetration of fertile men and that in infertile marriages (Ulstein 1972). A statistical correlation is, also, seen between the fertility of donors in artificial insemination, in vitro cervical penetration, and the duration of motility of spermatozoa in cervical mucus (Ulstein 1973). Glass wool filtration does not appear to affect the depth of penetration of 'normal' samples; however, when viscous samples are filtered, the statistically increased penetration and spermatozoal survival maintained for four hours demonstrates that column filtration yields healthier samples with better potential for fertilization.

The reported success rates aimed at improving spermatogenesis and the quality of the ejaculate remain unsatisfactory; therefore, many authors have tried to select, concentrate, preserve, and pool good spermatozoa from several ejaculates for later use in artifical insemination. Cryopreservation of semen in liquid nitrogen causes a significant impairment of spermatozoal viability with reduced conception rates (Behrman 1971; Sherman 1973). In vitro penetration of cervical mucus by sperm that has undergone cryopreservation and thawing is less than that of unfrozen spermatozoa (Fjallbrant and Ackerman 1973). By the use of filtration improvement in motility after freezing in liquid nitrogen and in cervical mucus penetration depth after cryopreservation potentially makes the samples more fertile.

Column filtration of samples with decreased sperm densities may further impair the count. Concentration of these ejaculates by centrifugation yields samples with good motility and sperm densities within the fertile range but with decreased volumes (Verdaquer et al. 1978). Concentration by centrifugation or by other methods being tested would allow for the potential to store several samples by cryopreservation for later inseminations. The addition of caffeine may or may not also improve the fertility potential of the ejaculate, whether the sample is to be used fresh or frozen.

3.2. Case studies

Three couples with infertility of at least two years duration had male partners with normal semen parameters except for decreased motility and increased residual viscosity after liquefaction. Artifical insemination utilizing glass wool filtered specimens was performed by application of a cervical cap (Comhaire and Vermeulen, 1978, unpublished). Pregnancy was obtained in two cases during the first insemination cycle and in one case during the third cycle.

Three other couples manifested increased sperm agglutination and repeatedly demonstrated no progressive motile spermatozoa six to ten hours after coitus in postcoital test. A shaking phenomenon was, also, observed during the sperm-cervical mucus contact test. Intrauterine insemination of 0.25 ml of filtered ejaculate was performed. Two women out of the three couples became pregnant. The first was an ectopic pregnancy after one cycle of insemination; the second couple conceived on the fourth cycle after four years of infertility – a normal child was delivered after a uneventful pregnancy.

4. LABORATORY APPLICATION

Approximately 35% of ejaculates used for antibody resting have either extremely high viscosity or a large amount of auto-agglutination of the spermatozoa. These ejaculates have presented technical problems and complications in the interpretation of the test results. Antibody tests comparing portions of samples before and after filtration to positive and negative controls reveal no immunological difference produced by column filtration (Paulson et al. 1978, 1979). This procedure can be utilized routinely for antibody testing, thereby decreasing technical and interpretational difficulties.

Research involving spermatozoal motility and its changes due to pharmacological substances, bacteria, bacterial filtrates, and other components is simplified if the great majority of spermatozoa is motile at the beginning of the experiment, since a large change in motility can thereby be produced, rather than the small one produced if the initial motility was only in the range of 50%. Studies have been performed using this technique and have proved encouraging for future research (Paulson and Polakoski, 1977c, 1977d).

REFERENCES

Amelar RD: *Infertility in men: diagnosis and treatment*, Philadelphia, Davis, 1966.
Barkay J, Zuckerman H, Sklan D, Gordon S: Effect of caffeine on increasing the motility of frozen human sperm. *Fertil Steril* 28: 175, 1977.
Behrman SJ: Preservation of human sperm by liquid nitrogen vapor freezing. In: *Current problems in fertility*, Ingelman-Sunberg A, Lunell NO (eds), New York, Plenum, 1971.
Bunge RG: Caffeine stimulation of ejaculated spermatozoa. *Urology* 1:371 (1973).
Fjallbrant B, Ackerman DR: Cervical mucus penetration in vitro by fresh and frozen-preserved human semen specimens. *J Reprod Fertil* 20:515, 1969.
Paulson JD, Polakoski KL: A glass wool column procedure for removing extraneous material from the human ejaculate. *Fertil Steril* 28:178, 1977a.
Paulson JD, Polakoski KL: Preparation of human semen by glass wool columns. In: *Techniques in human andrology*. Hafez ESE (ed), New York, Elsevier, 1977b.
Paulson JD, Polakoski KL: Isolation of a spermatozoal immobilization factor from Escherichia Coli filtrates. *Fertil Steril* 28:182, 1977c.
Paulson JD, Polakoski KL: Further characterization of the spermatozoal immobilization factor from Escherichia. *Fertil Steril* 28:315 1977d.
Paulson JD, Polakoski KL, Leto S: Further characterization of glass wool column filtration of human semen. *Fertil Steril* 32:125, 1979.
Paulson JD, Polakoski KL, Leto S: Glass wool column filtration. Presented at the first international symposium on AIH and male subfertility, Bordeaux, 1978.
Sherman JK: Synopsis of the use of frozen human semen since 1964: state of the art of human semen banking. *Fertil Steril* 24:397, 1973.
Ulstein M: Sperm penetration of cervical mucus as a criterion of male fertility. *Acta Obstet Gynecol Scand* 51:335, 1972.
Ulstein M: Fertility of donors at heterologous insemination. *Acta Obstet Gynecol Scand* 52:97, 1973.
Verdaquer S, Emperaire JC, Audebert A: Modifications du spermopris filtration sur laine de verre. Presented at the first international symposium on AIH and male subfertility, Bordeaux, 1978.

7. ADDITION OF PHARMACOLOGICAL AGENTS TO THE EJACULATE

J.D. Paulson, R. Harrison, W.B.Schill and J. Barkay

Knowledge of the anatomical mechanisms of sperm motility has come a long way from the homunculus theory suggested by Hartsoecker in 1698. Electron microscopic studies have shown that the motility of human spermatozoa is provided in the axial spiral complex of the tail (Pedersen 1970) by a sliding mechanism of the axonemal microtubules with respect to one another under the gripping action of the outer and inner dynein arms (Huxley 1969). This produces contractions and relaxations in the tail, propelling the spermatozoon in a quasi-purposeful manner, a self-propulsion that must suffice if it is to achieve contact with the released ovum after the initial extra impetus given by the neuromuscular movements of the male reproductive tract and the possible copulatory motor activity of the female genital tract have finished.

Immature spermatozoa are incapable of this self-propulsion and while this property, like fertilization capacity (Cooper and Orgebin-Crist 1975) is acquired in the epididymis (Gadden 1968), they only become truly motile on ejaculation. Motility is also affected adversely by the age of the man (MacLeod 1951), the morphology and length of time after ejaculation (Bartak 1971), certain sperma-tozoal shapes (Mitchell et al. 1976) and the part of the ejaculate in which the spermatozoon is extruded (Eliasson and Lindholmer 1972). External influences such as pH (Kroeks and Kremer 1977), temperature (Zaneveld and Polakoski 1977), ionic environment (Mitchell et al. 1976), light (van Duijn and van Lierop 1966), sources of irradiation (Norman et al. 1962) and the presence of antibodies (Fjallbrant 1968) may also affect motility. In addition abnormalities in the seminal plasma (Polakoski and Zaneveld 1977) or cervical mucus (Wolf et al. 1977) can be related to motility of the spermatozoa. A correlation has also been noted between sperm metabolism and concentration of zinc (Huacuja et al. 1973) and spermine (Fair et al. 1972).

Because of the many factors involved in and affecting the process of sperma-tozoal motility, an ejaculate with spermatozoa having abnormal motility but with other normal parameters may well benefit from the addition of some pharmacological agent to it in order to increase motility. This beneficial effect may allow insemination of a more motile specimen, thereby increasing the chance of pregnancy.

Several pharmacological agents have been utilized to increase motility in semen specimens in which there was poor movement. The substances are: (1) methylxanthines, (2) kinins, (3) L-arginine, and (4) prostaglandins.

1. PHARMACOLOGICAL AGENTS

1.1. Methylxanthines

Methylxanthines – caffeine, theophylline, and aminophylline – are inhibitors of phosphodiesterase. Addition of these substances in proper dosages may increase the concentration of cyclic AMP and cyclic GMP in spermatozoa (Figure 1). ATP, under the influence of adenylcyclase, is converted to cyclic AMP, which has been shown to stimulate human sperm motility (Hicks et al. 1972a). Because of the potential buildup of cyclic AMP and its known effect on spermatozoa it was felt that addition of a methylxanthine to the ejaculate would increase energy production by accelerating glycolysis and would therefore stimulate motility. Methylxanthines such as caffeine (1,3,7-trimethyl-2,6-dioxopurine) have been shown to stimulate metabolic activity of both epididymal (Drevius 1971) and ejaculated (Garbers et al. 1971) bull spermatozoa. The stimulatory effect was noted to be greater on the precapacitated specimens although motility is only progressive if seminal plasma is also present (Hoskins and Casillas 1975). Such metabolic effects could be modulated by alterations in the adenylcyclase-cyclic

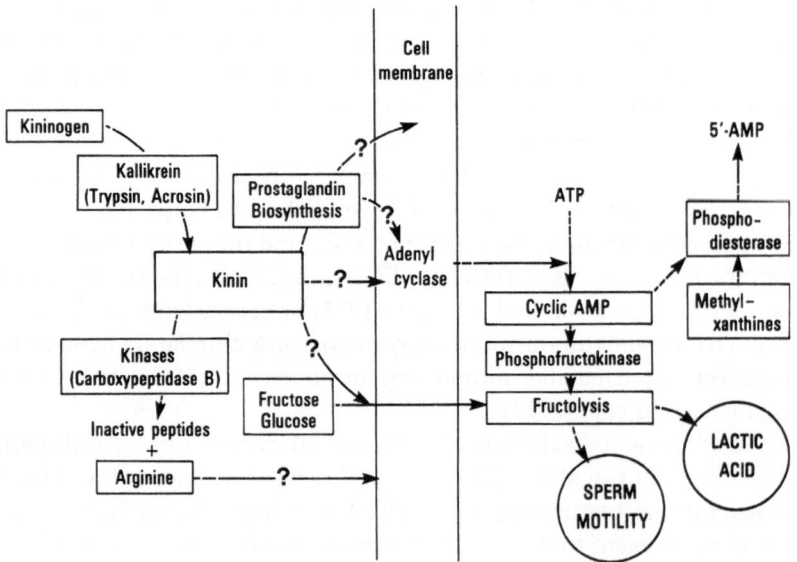

Figure 1. Possible mechanisms and interactions of various substances in relation to sperm motility.

AMP metabolic system, for caffeine is a cyclic nucleotide phosphodiesterase enzyme inhibitor (Hardman et al. 1971), and its addition could therefore influence cyclic nucleotide concentrations with a consequent alteration in spermatozoal metabolism and motility.

The addition of caffeine to the human semen in a final concentration of approximately 6mMol not only stimulated a greater number of ejaculatory spermatozoa to become motile but increased the rate of motility and forward progression of the sperm (Bunge 1973; Haesungcharern and Chulavatnatol 1973); Schoenfeld et al. 1973, 1975). The addition of caffeine to cryopreserved specimens has also been shown to stimulate motility (Barkay et al. 1977).

Harrison (1978) noted significant stimulation of spermatozoal motility in 34 patients, 14 of whom had semen analyses within normal limits, using the same dosage regimen as previously described. These specimens were then artificially inseminated. The results were validated by comparison with placebo (Modified Ringer's solution), each patient acting as her own control. Four hundred inseminations were carried out (199 with caffeine-enhanced semen); however, only one pregnancy ensued, and that in a patient inseminated with semen plus placebo.

1.2. Kinins

Kinins are polypeptides produced through an enzymatic breakdown of a precursor substrate kininogen, by a kininogenase (kallikrein), a proteolytic enzyme present in tissue. Kinins are potent pharmacologically and in very low doses have the ability to cause vasodilation, leading to a lowering of blood pressure. They are also able to increase capillary permeability, produce edema and pain and contract or relax different smooth muscles, including the uterus and small bowel. The factors involved in the formation and destruction of the kallikrein-kinin system are not dissimilar in form from those of coagulation, fibrolysis, and the complement system (Figure 1). All components of this mechanism are present in the male and female genital secretions (Palm et al. 1976; Schill and Preissler 1977) and continuous production and destruction of kinins occurs as long as kininogen, kinin-liberating proteinases (kallikrein) and kinin-inactivating enzymes are present. Acrosin, as well as trypsin and a kininogenase from the prostate, has the ability to liberate kinins from kininogen (Palm and Fritz 1975). This proteolytic enzyme which allows penetration of the zona pellucida is known to be present in the acrosome of the spermatozoa and is in an enzyme-inhibitor complex and zymogen form in the seminal plasma (Fritz et al. 1975; Polakoski et al. 1977). The possibility exists that as the spermatozoa penetrate through cervical mucus, acrosin might be released, thereby liberating kinins.

Addition of hog pancreatic kallikrein to semen samples with sperm motilities between 25% and 50% causes an increase in sperm motility, not only in the total number of motile spermatozoa, but also in the number of progressively moving spermatozoa (Schill et al. 1974; Leidl et al. 1975; Schirren 1975; Wallner et al. 1975; Steiner et al. 1977; Schill and Haberland 1974a). An increase in the mean velocity (Steiner et al. 1977) and a small improvement in the viability (Leidl et al. 1975) of the samples have also been noted. The spermatozoa show an increased metabolic state indicated by an increase in fructolysis (Schill 1975a), increased oxygen consumption (Leidl et al. 1975), increased lactic acid and CO_2 production (Leidl et al. 1975; Schill et al. 1975) and increased intracellular cyclic AMP levels (Schill and Preissler 1977). The effect on semen samples by kallikrein was also seen in ejaculates that were 24 hours old (Schill 1975b), as well as samples that were cryopreserved (Schill et al. 1976; Schill and Pritsch 1976; Schill 1977). The effects of kallikrein can be inhibited by the trypsin-kallikrein inhibitor from bovine organs (Trasylol ®, from Bayer A.G.) or inactivated by acid denaturation, demonstrating that the increase in sperm motility seen by addition of kallikrein can be attributed to its enzymatic properties as a kinin-releasing proteinase (Schill 1975d). A direct stimulatory effect of sperm motility by addition of bradykinin and kallidin is observed to last between one and two hours (Schill 1975b). The shorter duration of increased spermatozoal motility by kinins in comparison to kallikrein is probably a direct effect of the kinases on the kinins in the seminal plasma, in comparison to the longer effect of increased motility with the addition of kallikrein due to a constant liberation of kinins from kininogen for a long time interval. Addition of carboxypeptidase-B, a potent kinase, decreases motility of the spermatozoa in ejaculates with good semen quality (Schill and Haberland 1974b). The kallikrein-kinin system may therefore regulate and stimulate sperm motility.

In vitro cervical mucus penetration has been shown to correlate significantly with conception indices and fertilizing ability (Ulstein 1972, 1973). Significant improvement of spermatozoal in vitro cervical mucus penetration can be observed on the addition of pancreatic kallikrein (Wallner et al. 1975; Schill et al. 1976; Schill and Preissler 1977). When aprotinin (Trasylol ®), a kallikrein inhibitor was added, the effect of the increased cervical mucus penetration by the addition of kallikrein was negated. The effect of kinins (bradykinin) was seen to be similar to that of kallikrein in their ability to stimulate oligospermic semen specimens with increased cervical mucus penetration. The effect was also seen to be a direct one, rather than being due to activation of a mediator system.

1.2.1. Caffeine and kinin: a comparison. The addition of caffeine and kallikrein to different portions of the same ejaculate demonstrated different changes in sperm motility (Schill 1975c). Caffeine induces an immediate increase in sperm motility, this effect remaining relatively constant during the first several hours; however by 24 hours the caffeine-treated samples demonstrate the same motility as untreated controls. Kallikrein's effect of increasing sperm motility is delayed, with maximum stimulation at two hours. Adding both caffeine and kallikrein simultaneously to a sample further increases the motility of the spermatozoa significantly over that produced by either alone.

Caffeine and kallikrein added after thawing to cryopreserved samples in final concentrations of 5mMol and 5KU/ml (KU = kallikrein unit) respectively demonstrated a significant improvement over the post-thaw total motility by an increase of 81% with caffeine and 73% with kallikrein after one hour of incubation (Schill et al. 1979). A similar pattern of 80% increase with caffeine and 54% increase in the presence of kallikrein was observed after incubating for four hours. The simultaneous addition of both substances was significantly better than either agent alone and demonstrated an average increase of 119% (Figure 2) after one hour and 114% after four hours. Forward progressive motility was also improved by the addition of both caffeine and kallikrein. As with the total motility, the best stimulation of forward progressive motility was obtained by the simultaneous addition of both substances to the cryopreserved thawed specimens (Figure 3). The metabolism of the cryopreserved specimens was investigated utilizing fructolysis. There was a significant increase in fructolysis after four hours of incubation in the presence of caffeine. Kallikrein however showed a statistically significant increase in fructose utilization only after 24 hours (Schill et al. 1978).

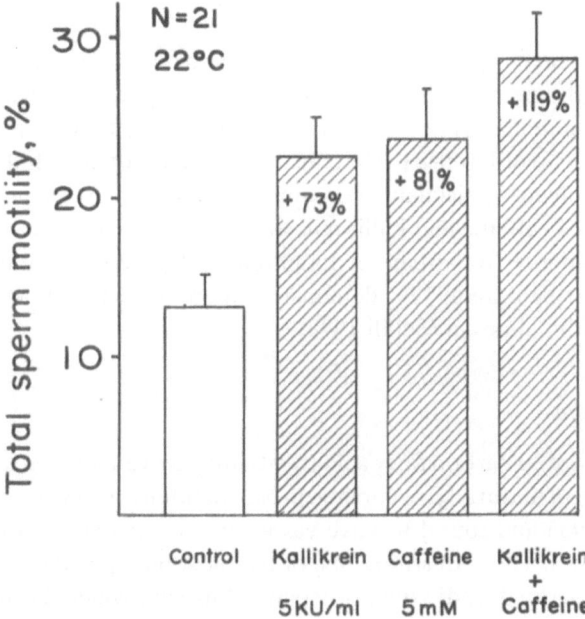

Figure 2. The total motility of 21 cryopreserved thawed ejaculates after the addition of kallikrein, caffeine, or both (incubation time 1 hour).

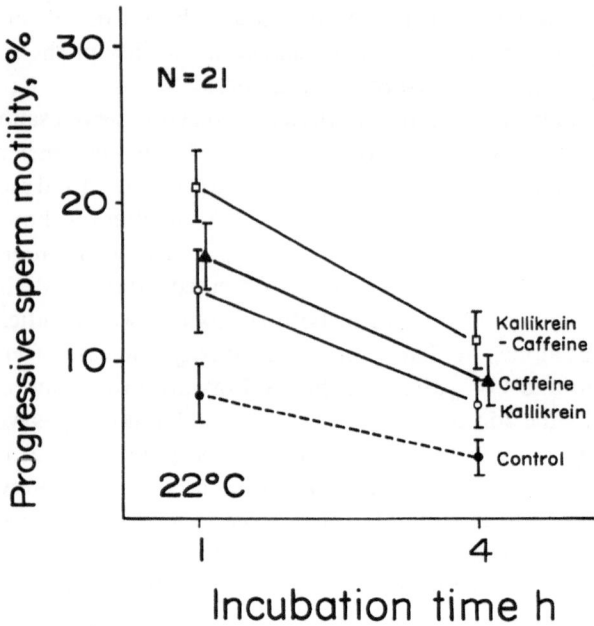

Figure 3. Progressive motility of 21 cryopreserved thawed ejaculates over a 4-hour time interval after the addition of caffeine, kallikrein, or both.

Initial cervical mucus penetration depth by sperm was improved by the addition of either caffeine or kallikrein. Significant increased penetration was obtained by the simultaneous addition of both substances. However after a two-hour time period, no difference to the controls could be noted (Schill et al. 1978).

In a study involving 57 ejaculates containing hypokinetic spermatozoa (Figure 4), the addition of caffeine and kallikrein to these specimens demonstrated that 40% had no response to caffeine or kallikrein; 39% showed stimulation with either caffeine or kallikrein; 12% demonstrated an increase only with caffeine; and 9% only with kallikrein (Schill 1978).

1.3. Prostaglandins

Prostaglandins are 20-carbon fatty acids containing a five-membered ring. There are five groups of naturally occurring prostaglandins, which were originally discovered in 1933 and found to have vasodepressor and smooth muscle contracting properties. They constitute one of the most biologically active types of compounds discovered. Individual prostaglandins vary widely both in potency and in their activities.

Prostaglandin-E levels decrease in infertile males (Bygdeman et al. 1970; Hawkins 1967; Collier et al. 1975). Prostaglandin-F2α added to semen speci-

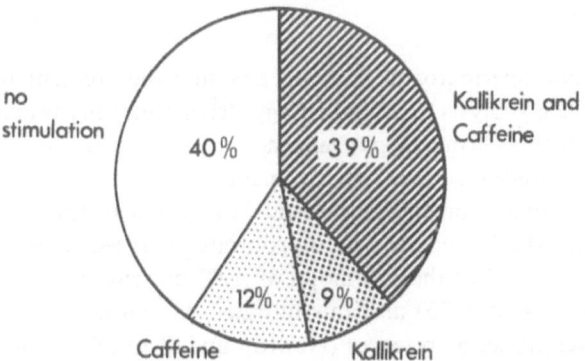

Figure 4. The percentage of 57 ejaculates demonstrating stimulation of motility after the addition of caffeine or kallikrein (Schill 1978).

mens in concentrations one hundred times greater than found in normal semen resulted in significant inhibition of sperm motility (Cohen et al. 1977). In contrast, addition of physiologic levels of prostaglandin-F2α to spermatozoa increased in vitro penetration into cervical mucus (Eskin et al. 1973). It has also been found by other investigators (Hunt and Zaneveld 1975) that the time required for spermatozoal penetration of cervical mucus was greatly diminished by the addition of small doses of prostaglandins-F1α or F2α. The addition of prostaglandin-E was less effective.

1.4. L-arginine

L-arginine is a non-essential aminoacid found in seminal plasma. It has been demonstrated that acrosin, the proteolytic enzyme at the head of the sperm, preferentially catalyzes the hydrolysis of arginine substrates (Paulson et al. 1979). Kinases cleave the carboxy-terminal arginine from kinins yielding arginine and inactive peptides. A clinical report of oral arginine treatment of oligospermic males with subsequent successes (Schachter et al. 1973) spurred an interest in this aminoacid as a possible therapeutic treatment for oligospermia. Others, however, were not able to reproduce the improved results (Jungling and Bunge 1976). In vitro testing was performed by the addition of L-arginine in a final concentration of 4mMol (Keller and Polakoski 1975). The average increase of forward motile spermatozoa was 82% compared with controls. Other aminoacids, although both similar in structure and arginine analogs (D-arginine. L-nitroarginine, L-homoarginine, L-lysine and L-ornithine) were not effective in stimulation.

2. PHYSIOLOGY

Although human spermatozoa have an absolute requirement for exogenous hexoses to drive glycolysis, the final energy-driving motility is chiefly provided internally, with the plasma membrane helping to control and modulate the effects that the differing external environments have on the process. This energy source is ATP situated on the mitochondria adjacent to the axial spiral complex. Ca^{++} and Mg^{++} mediate the appropriate ATP ase activity metabolism (enzymatic hydrolysis) of the 150 moles of ATP present in each spermatozoon (Petersen and Freund 1973) and this initiates the tail motion. Other organic phosphates present act as reserves (Newton and Rothschild 1961). Some oxidative metabolism does occur (Petersen and Freund 1973), involving the cyclic AMP system (Hicks et al. 1972b); and endogenous respiratory activity, perhaps derived from the oxidation of intracellular phospho-lipids (Mann 1964; Poulos and White 1973), can support motility (Nevo 1966). However ATP levels soon become depleted and all motility ceases within a few hours unless fructose becomes involved in the regeneration of ATP (Petersen and Freund 1970). The metabolism is however chiefly glycolytic, with minimal oxygen consumption, and most hexoses that are consumed by the human spermatozoa appear in the suspending medium as lactic acid, whether or not there has been oxygen present (MacLeod and Freund 1958). This pathway in the human appears to be under the influence of nucleotide phosphodiesterase enzymes (Hicks et al. 1972a), the release of which is inhibited by high ATP levels. Therefore, as these levels are used up, the enzymes become released with resultant increase in glycolysis (Atkinson and Walton 1967). The natural activators of this mechanism remain to be identified but a role for cyclic AMP related to capacitation has been noted in rabbits (Rosado et al. 1974). Higher levels of AMP increase enzyme activation. Cyclic AMP appears to bind on the surface of the membrane of the attached spermatozoa (Rosado et al. 1976) and the amount present appears to be directly related to this spermatozoal activity (Tash and Mann 1973), which would suggest that the amount present appears to be directly related to this spermatozoal activity of the cyclic nucleotides (Cyclic AMP and GMP) which are intimately connected with sperm metabolism, acting from exogenous and endogenous sources during the spermatozoal life cycle in its passage from testis to fallopian tube.

   The observations of the different responses of the motility of the ejaculates to the addition of caffeine and kallikrein in fresh (Schill 1975c) and cryopreserved thawed specimens (Schill et al. 1979) and the utilization of fructose in these samples (Schill et al. 1979) indicate differences in the mode of action of the two systems. Simultaneous addition of both substances led to further improvement of sperm motility over and above either alone (Schill 1975; Schill et al. 1978). Although there is an increase in intracellular cyclic AMP levels after stimulation by the kinin system (Schill and Preissler 1977), the amount is small and it is, therefore, doubtful that the kinins increase sperm motility in the same manner as the methylxanthines, which stimulate via the inhibition of phosphodiesterase and the buildup of cyclic AMP (Figure 1). The mode of stimulation of sperm motility by kinins is still unknown. An effect of kinins on prostaglandin synthesis has been suggested (Damas and Deby 1974; Ferreira et al. 1974). It has been demonstrated that when mefenamate, a potent inhibitor of prostaglandin synthesis (in vitro) was added to an ejaculate, the kallikrein-kinin effect on sperm motility and oxygen consumption was inhibited (Gryglewski 1974). However, the addition of prostaglandins to the ejaculate containing mefenamate and kallikrein restored and increased the motility. It is also mechanistically possible that kinins help facilitate transport of hexoses into the cell.

In addition to their relationship with the kinin system, prostaglandins have been shown to interact with other systems. Although caffeine-induced stimulation of sperm motility is thought to be due to its action as an inhibitor of phosphodiesterase with subsequent buildup of cyclic AMP, it has been shown that caffeine will inhibit prostaglandin-15-dehydrogenase (Marrazzi and Matschinsky 1972), an important enzyme in the degradation of prostaglandins.

There is also strong evidence that prostaglandins produce their actions as part of an interaction with the cyclic AMP system (Ramwell and Shaw 1971), and in most systems prostaglandin-E has been accepted as a strong stimulus for accumulation of cyclic AMP (Marsh and LeMaire 1974).

The mechanism of the effect of in vitro L-arginine addition remains unresolved. L-arginine is a non-essential aminoacid and theoretically there should be no in vivo shortage of it; however, it has been demonstrated that the concentration of arginine in men with normal sperm counts is greater than that in oligospermic and aspermic individuals (Krampitz and Doepfmer 1962). From in vitro studies (Keller and Polakoski 1975) it appears that the terminal guanidine group as well as the chain length of the aminoacid are necessary for its action.

The fact that in vitro addition of caffeine and subsequent insemination failed to improve pregnancy rates is disappointing (Harrison 1978). These results plus the findings of others (Dougherty et al. 1976; Schill 1978) that effects of methylxanthines and kinins are not uniform in all semen specimens suggest that especially where semen samples are already poor, these substances may not really make samples as 'normal' as they apparently become. Instead they may in some way damage spermatozoa whose normality is perhaps already in doubt, thus preventing fertilization. Indeed, changes have been noted in morphology on caffeine-enhanced semen (Harrison and Sheppard 1978, unpublished). There may, however, be other reasons for such results as it has been recorded (Barkay and Zuckerman 1978) that adding caffeine to specimens prior to cryopreservation has produced no adverse effect on fertility rates, although is must be assumed that such semen is obviously impeccable in quality from the beginning. Our knowledge and understanding of the metabolism of human spermatozoa is still incomplete. The natural activators in the metabolic systems in spermatozoa remain to be identified. The site of action of the interaction between motility and capacitation are as yet incompletely understood and much knowledge has been applied from experimental animal data, which does not always apply to humans. It is, therefore, not surprising that the addition of compounds to semen does not always appear to produce the desired effects. However, although addition of these compounds to human semen cannot yet be recommended, experimental pursuits may yet prove to be most rewarding, enabling effective forms of therapy to be devised for the infertile male – therapy based on accepting and treating the seminal sample that can actually be produced rather than trying to get a damaged gonad to perform better.

REFERENCES

Atkinson EE, Walton GE: Adenosine triphosphate concentration in metabolic regulation. *J Biol Chem* 242:3239, 1967.
Barkay J, Zuckerman H: Paper presented at the first international symposium on AIH and male subfertility. Bordeaux, 1978.
Barkay J, Zuckerman H: Paper presented at the first international symposium on AIH and male subfertility. Bordeaux, 1978.
Bartak V: Sperm velocity test in clinical practice. *Int J Fertil* 16:107, 1971.
Behrman SJ: Preservation of human sperm by liquid nitrogen vapor freezing. In: *Current problems in fertility*, Ingelman-Sundberg A, Lunell NO (eds), New York, Plenum, 1971.
Behrman SJ, Ackerman DR:Freeze preservation of human spermatozoa. *Am J Obstet Gynecol* 103:654, 1969.
Bunge RG: Caffeine stimulation of ejaculated human spermatozoa. *Urology* 1:371, 1973.
Bygdeman M: Prostaglandins in human seminal fluid and their correlation to fertility. *Int J Fertil* 14:228, 1969.
Bygdeman M, Fredricsson B, Svanborg K, Samuelsson B: The relation between fertility and prostaglandin content of seminal fluid in man. *Fertil Steril* 21:622, 1970.
Cohen MS, Colin MJ, Golimbu M, Hotchkiss RS: The effects of prostaglandins on sperm motility. *Fertil Steril* 28:78, 1977.
Collier JG, Flower RJ, Stanton SL: Seminal prostaglandins in infertile men. *Fertil Steril* 26:868, 1975.
Cooper TG, Orgebin-Crist MD: The effect of epididiymal and testicular fluid on the fertilizing capacity of testicular and epididymal spermatozoa. *Andrologia* 7: 85, 1975.
Damas J, Deby C: Libération de prostaglandines par la bradykinine chez le rat. *C R Soc Biol* 168:375, 1974.
Dougherty KA, Cockett A, Urry R: Caffeine, Theophylline, and human sperm motility. *Fertil Steril* 27:541, 1976.
Drevius LO: The sperm rise test. *J Reprod Fert* 24:427, 1971.
Duijn C van, Lierop JH van: Effect of temperature on photosensitivity of spermatozoa. *Nature* 201:5055, 1966.
Eliasson R, Lindholmer C: Distribution and properties of spermatozoa in different fractions of split ejaculates. *Fertil Steril* 23:252, 1972.
Eskin BA, Azarbal S, Sepic R, Slate WG: In vitro responses of the spermatozoa-cervical mucus system treated with prostaglandin-F2α. *Obstet Gynecol* 41:436, 1973.

Fair W, Clarke R, Wehner N: A correlation of seminal polyamine levels and semen analysis in the human. *Fertil Steril* 23:38, 1972.

Ferreira SH, Moncada S, Vane JR: Prostaglandins and signs and symptoms of inflammation. In: *Prostaglandin synthetase inhibitors*, Robinson HJ, Vane JR (eds). New York, Raven, 1974, p 175.

Fjallbrant B: Interrelation between high levels of sperm antibodies, reduced penetration of cervical mucus by spermatozoa and sterility in men. *Acta Obstet Synecol Scand* 47:102, 1968.

Fjallbrant B, Ackerman DR: Cervical mucus penetration in vitro by fresh and frozen-preserved human semen specimens, *J Reprod Fertil* 20:515, 1969.

Fritz H, Schiessler H, Schill WB, Tscheache H, Heimburger N, Wallner O: Low molecular weight proteinase (acrosin) inhibitors from human and boar seminal plasma and spermatozoa and human cervical mucus: isolation, properties, and biological aspects. In: *Proteases and biological control*, Reich E, Rifkin DB, Shaw E (eds), Cold Spring Harbor Laboratory, 1975.

Gadden P: Sperm maturation in the male reproductive tract: development of motility. *Anat Rec* 161:471, 1968.

Garbers DL, First NL, Sullivan JT, Lardy HA: Stimulation and maintenance of ejaculated bovine spermatozoa respiration and motility by caffeine. *Biol Reprod* 5:336, 1971.

Gryglewski RJ: Structure-activity relationships of some prostaglandin synthetase inhibitors. In: *Prostaglandin synthetase inhibitors*, Robinson HJ, Vane JR (eds), New York, Raven, 1974, p 33.

Haesungcharern A, Chulavatnatol M: Stimulation of human spermatozoal motility by caffeine. *Fertil Steril* 27:662, 1973.

Hardman JG, Robinson GA, Sutherland EW: Cyclic nucleotides. *Annual Review of Physiol* 33:331, 1971.

Harrison RF: Insemination of husband's semen with and without addition of caffeine. *Fertil Steril* 29:532, 1978.

Hawkins DF: In: *Symposium of the Worcester foundation for experimental biology*, Ramwell PW, Shaw JE (eds), New York, Interscience, 1967, p. 1.

Hicks JJ, Pedron N, Martinez-Manautoi J, Rodado A: Metabolic changes in human spermatozoa related to capacitation. *Fertil Steril* 23:172, 1972a.

Hicks JJ, Pedron N, Rosado A: Modifications of human spermatozoa glycolysis by cyclic adenosine monophosphate (CAMP), estrogens and follicular fluid. *Fertil Steril* 23:886, 1972b.

Hoskins DD, Casillas ER: Function of cyclic nucleotides in mammalian spermatozoa. In: *Handbook of physiology*, volume 5, section 7: *Endocrinology of the reproductive system: male*, Greepro L, Astwood EB (eds), Washington DC, American Physiological Society, 1975.

Huacuja L, Sosa A, Delgrado NM, Rosado A: Kinetic study of the participation of zinc in human spermatozoa metabolism. *Life Sci* 13:1383, 1973.

Hunt WL, Zaneveld LJD: Prostaglandin effects on sperm penetration of cervical mucus. Abstract 31, international conference of andrology, Detroit, 1975.

Huxley HE: Mechanism of muscular contraction. *Science* 164:1356, 1969.

Jungling ML, Bunge RG: The treatment of spermatogenic arrest with arginine. *Fertil Steril* 27:282, 1976.

Keller DW, Polakoski KL: L-arginine stimulation of human sperm motility in vitro. *Biol Reprod* 13:154, 1975.

Krampitz G, Doepfmer, R: Determination of free amino-acids in human ejaculate by ion exchange chromatography. *Nature* 194:684, 1962.

Kroeks M, Kremer J: The pH in the lower third of the genital tract. In: *The uterine cervix in reproduction*, Insler V, Bettendorf G, Stuttgart, Georg Thieme, 1977, p 109.

Leidl W, Prinzen R, Schill W-B, Fritz H: The effect of kallikrein on motility and metabolism of spermatozoa in vitro. In: *Kininogenases, kallikrein: second symposium on physiological properties and pharmacological rationale*, Haberland GL, Rohen JW, Schirren C, Huber P (eds), Stuttgart, Schattauer, 1975, p 33.

MacLeod J: Semen quality in 1,000 men of known fertility and 800 of infertile marriages. *Fertil Steril* 2:115, 1951.

MacLeod J, Freund M: Influence of spermatozoa concentration and initial fructose level on fructolysis of human semen. *J Appl Physiol* 13:501, 1958.

Mann T: *Biochemistry of semen and of the male reproductive tract* (2nd edition), New York, John Wiley and Sons, 1964.

Marrazzi MA, Matschinsky M: Properties of 15-hydroxyprostaglandin dehydrogenase: structural requirements for binding *Prostaglandins* 1:373, 1972.

Marsh JM, LeMaire WJ: Cyclic AMP accumulation and steroidogenesis in the human corpus luteum: effect of gonadotropins and prostaglandins. *J. Clin Endocrinol Metab* 39:99, 1974.

Mitchell J, Nelson L, Hafez ESE: Motility of spermatozoa. In: *Human semen infertility regulation in men*, Hafez ESE (ed), St. Louis, Mosby, 1976.

Nevo A: Relations between motility and respiration in human spermatozoa. *Rep Fert* 16:351, 1966.

Newton AA, Rothschild L: Energy-rich phosphate compounds in bull semen: comparison of their metabolism with anaerobic heat production and impedance change frequency. *Proc Royal Soc Lond (Biol)* 155:183, 1961.

Norman C, Goldberg E, Porterfield I: The effect of visible radiation on the functional life span of mammalian and avian sperm. *Exp Cell Res* 28:69, 1962.

Palm S, Fritz H: Kinases in cervical mucus and seminal plasma. In: *Kininogenases, Kallekrein, second symposium on physiological properties and pharmacological rationale*, Haberland GL, Rohen JW, Schirren C, Huber P (eds), Stuttgart, Schattauer, 1975.

Palm S, Schill, W-B, Wallner O, Prinzen R, Fritz H: Occurrence of components of the kallikrein-kinin system in human genital tract secretions and their possible function in stimulation of sperm motility and migration. In: *Kinins: pharmacodynamics and biological roles*, Sicuteri F, Back A, Haberland GL (eds), New York, Plenum, 1976, p. 271.

Paulson JD, Parrish RF, Polakowski KL: Comparative synthetic substrate kinetics of porcine acrosin and porcine β-trypsin. *Int J Bio* 10:247, 1979.

Pedersen H: Observations of the axial filament complex of the human spermatozoon. *J Ultrastructures* 33:451, 1970.

Petersen RN, Freund M: ATP synthesis and oxidative metabolism in human spermatozoa. *Biol Reprod* 3:47, 1970.

Petersen RN, Freund M: Effects of H^+ and certain membrane-active drugs on glycolysis, motility and ATP *Biol Reprod* 8:350, 1973.

Polakoski K, Zaneveld L: Biochemical examination of the human ejaculate. In: *Techniques of human andrology*, Hafez ESE (ed), Amsterdam, North-Holland Biomedical Press, 1977, p 265.

Polakoski KL, Zahler WL, Paulson JD: Demonstration of proacrosin and quantitation of acrosin in ejaculated human spermatozoa. *Fertil Steril* 28:688, 1977.

Poulos A, White I: Phospholipid composition of human spermatozoa and seminal plasma. *J Reprod Fertil* 35:265, 1973.

Ramwell P, Shaw H: The biological significance of the prostaglandins. *Ann N Y Acad Sci* 180:10, 1970.

Rosado A, Hicks JJ, Reyes A, Blanco J: Capacitation in vitro of rabbit spermatozoa with cyclic adenosine monophosphate and human follicular fluid. *Fertil Steril* 25:82, 1974.

Rosado A, Huacuja L, Delgardo N, Pancardo R: Cyclic AMP receptors in the human spermatozoa membrane. *Life Sci* 17:1707, 1976.

Schachter A, Goldman JA, Zuckerman Z: Treatment of oligospermia with the amino acid arginine. *J Urol* 110:311, 1973.

Schill W-B: Humane Spermakonservierung und therapeutische Ausblicke. *Hautarzt* 23:525, 1972.

Schill W-B: Increased fructolysis of kallikrein-stimulated human spermatozoa. *Andrologia* 7:105, 1975a.

Schill W-B: Stimulation of sperm motility by kinins in fresh and 24 hours aged human ejaculates. *Andrologia* 7:135, 1975b.

Schill W-B: Caffeine and kallikrein-induced stimulation of human sperm motility: a comparative study. *Andrologia* 7:229, 1975c.

Schill W-B: Influence of the kallikrein-kinin system on human sperm motility in vitro. In: *Kininogenase, second symposium on physiological properties and pharmacological rationale, kallikrein* Haberland GL, Rohen JW, Schirren C, Huber P (eds), Stuttgart, Schattauer, 1975d.

Schill W-B: Kallikrein as a therapeutical means in the treatment of male infertility. In: *Kininogenases, fourth symposium on physiological properties and pharmacological rationale, kallikrein:* Haberland GL, Rohen JW, Suzuki T (eds), Stuttgart, Schattauer, 1977, p 251.

Schill W-B: Effect of kallikrein on the motility of fresh and frozen human semen. Presented to the first international symposium on AIH and male subfertility, Bordeaux, 1978.

Schill W-B, Haber land GL: Kinin-induced enhancement of sperm motility. *Hoppe-Seyler's Z Physiol Chem* 355:299, 1974a.

Schill W-B, Haberland GL: In vitro stimulation of human sperm motility by kallikrein. *World Cong Fertil Steril* 8:153, 1974b.

Schill W-B, Preissler G: Improvement of cervical mucus spermatozoal penetration by kinins: a possible therapeutical approach in the treatment of male subfertility. In: *The uterine cervix in reproduction,* Insler V, Bettendorf G (eds), Stuttgart, Georg Thieme, 1977, p 134.

Schill W-B, Pritsch W: Kinin-induced enhancement of sperm motility in cryo-preserved human spermatozoa. *Proc Int Congress Animal Reprod Artif insemination* 8:1071, 1976.

Schill W-B, Pritsch W, Preissler G: Effect of caffeine and kallikrein on cryopreserved human spermatozoa. *Int J Fertil* 24:27, 1979.

Schill W-B, Braun-Falco O, Haberland GL: The possible role of kinins in sperm motilities. *Int J Fertil* 19:163, 1974.

Schill W-B, Leidl W, Prinzen R, Wallner O: Stimulation of sperm motility and sperm metabolism by kallikrein, a kinin-liberating proteinase. *Proc European Sterility Congres* 4:375, 1975.

Schill W-B, Wallner O, Palm S, Fritz H: Kinin stimulation of spermatozoa motility and migration in cervical mucus. In: *Human semen and fertility regulation in men,* Hafez ESE (ed), St. Louis Mosby, 1976, p 442.

Schirren C: Experimental studies on the influence of kallikrein on human sperm motility in vitro. In:*Kininoginases, kallikrein: second symposium on physiological properties and pharmacological rationale,* Haberland GL, Rohen JW, Schirren C, Huber P (eds), Stuttgart, Schattauer 1975, p 59.

Schoenfeld C, Amelar RD, Dubin L: Stimulation of ejaculated human spermatozoa by caffeine: a preliminary report. *Fertil Steril* 24:772, 1973.

Schoenfeld C, Amelar RD, Dubin L: Stimulation of ejaculated human spermatozoa by caffeine. *Fertil Steril* 26:158, 1975.

Sherman JK: Synopsis of the use of frozen human semen since 1964: state of the art of human semen banking. *Fertil Steril* 24:397, 1973.

Steiner R, Hofmann N, Hartmann R: The influence of kallikrein on the velocity of human spermatozoa measured by Laser-Doppler spectroscopy. In: *Kininogenases, kallikrein: fourth symposium on physiological properties and pharmacological rationale,* Haberland GL, Rohen JW, Suzuki T (eds), Stuttgart, Schattauer, 1977, p 229.

Tash JA, Mann FRC: Adenosine 3' 5' cyclic monophosphate in relation to motility and senescence of spermatozoa. *Proc Royal Soc Lond (Biol)* 184:109, 1973.

Ulstein M: Sperm penetration of cervical mucus as a criterion of male fertility. *Acta Obstet Gynecol Scand* 51:335, 1972.

Ulstein M: Fertility of donors at heterologous insemination. *Acta Obstet Gynecol Scand* 52:97, 1973.

Wallner O, Schill W-B, Brosser A, Fritz H: Participation of the kallikrein-kinin system in sperm penetration through cervical mucus: in vitro studies. In: *Kininogenases, kallikrein: second symposium on physiological properties and pharmacological rationale,* Haberland GL. Rohen JW, Schirren C, Huber P (eds), Stuttgart, Schattauer, 1975, p 63.

Wolf P, Blasco L, Khan MA, Litt M: Human Cervical mucus II: changes in viscoelasticity during the ovulatory menstrual cycle. *Fertil Steril* 28:47, 1977.

Zaneveld L, Polakoski K: Collection and the physical examination of the ejaculate. In: *Techniques in human andrology,* Hafez ESE (ed), Amsterdam, North-Holland Biomedical Press, 1977, p 159.

8. USE OF ALBUMIN COLUMNS FOR SEMEN FILTRATION IN MALE INFERTILITY

W.P. Dmowski, R.J. Ericsson, K.H. Broer and G.B. Carruthers

1. THE ROLE OF SEMEN FILTRATION PROCEDURES IN MALE INFERTILITY

The male factor is the cause of infertility or plays a significant contributory role in a large proportion of childless couples. It has been estimated that decreased sperm count and/or low motility occur among 40-50% of husbands in such couples (Speroff et al. 1978). The severity of the problem is reflected in the semen analysis, which may indicate absolute sterility, as in patients with azoospermia, or a relatively minor problem as in patients with mild oligospermia. In the semen of the majority of subfertile men, morphologically normal, motile spermatozoa are present, although in a significantly decreased number. Semen analysis in such cases usually reveals predominance of non-motile and abnormally formed spermatozoa, immature germ cells, germinal epithelium, leukocytes and other inflammatory cells, epithelial cells originating from excretory ducts or accessory sex organs, amorphous material, as well as other cellular and non-cellular debris. It is only infrequently that disorders such as endocrine disturbances, chromosomal abnormalities, varicocele, or infection can be identified as the cause of male infertility. In the majority of men with oligospermia or decreased motility no definite cause can be demonstrated.

To increase the percentage of morphologically normal, motile spermatozoa in the semen of infertile men two therapeutic approaches may potentially be of value. One involves a nonspecific hormonal treatment, not intended to correct identifiable etiologic factors, but rather aimed at stimulating spermatogenesis. The results are variable and generally unpredictable. If spermatogenesis improves, an increase in sperm density without change in the percentage of abnormal and non-motile spermatozoa may be observed.

The other therapeutic approach deals with the ejaculate. Chemical substances are added to the semen to increase the percentage of motile spermatozoa or the semen is processed in vitro, to isolate the morphologically normal motile fraction prior to the artificial, homologous insemination (AIH). A significant correlation has been demonstrated between the cumulative probability of pregnancy and the percentages of live spermatozoa and normal spermatozoa in the husband's semen (Eliasson 1971). No relationship was found, on the other hand, between the probability of pregnancy and the concentration of spermatozoa. It may be assumed, therefore, that separation of motile, morphologically normal spermatozoa from the abnormal forms and debris prior to AIH should improve the chances for conception.

Using various in vitro filtration procedures, abnormal and non-motile spermatozoa can be removed more or less efficiently along with seminal debris, while the percentage of morphologically normal, motile forms generally increases in the isolated fraction. Seminal plasma, which in some cases may contain factors suppressing the motility and vitality of spermatozoa (Syner et al. 1975), or which may contain bacteria and inflammatory cells from infected accessory sex organs, is usually removed with most of such procedures.

A variety of techniques for sperm separation prior to AIH have been reported, claiming varying rates of success in improving semen quality and in facilitating conception. A simple, natural form of sperm separation through collection of different fractions of the ejaculate, the so-called split ejaculate, has been widely used in clinical practice with reasonably good results. The fraction rich in spermatozoa (usually the first) is identified and used for AIH. Pregnancies have been achieved with this procedure when repeated attempts at insemination with the whole ejaculate had been unsuccessful (Amelar and Hotchkiss 1965; Farris and Murphy 1960; Kleegman and Kaufman 1966; Tyler 1961). Most of the seminal plasma is separated from spermatozoa with this method. The technique has been considered of value especially in patients with inflammatory processes in the accessory sex organs. But though a concentrated semen specimen can be obtained with this technique, there is no change in the percentage of abnormal spermatozoa and little change in motility and the amount of sperm debris. A form of split ejaculation that could be practiced during intercourse by the infertile couple without help of the physician has been recommended and success with this method has been claimed (Amelar and Dubin 1975).

The literature abounds with reports on in vitro techniques designed to separate normal from abnormal spermatozoa in subfertile husbands prior to AIH. A variety of physical separation methods such as filtration, centrifugation, washing and pooling, and chromatography have been reported with variable claims of success, but generally with little or no reproducibility. Most techniques are complicated; their results have been erratic in the hands of different investigators; and none has been generally accepted.

Two methods reported recently deserve more attention. Both techniques claim in vitro effectiveness in the isolation of motile spermatozoa and both have had some degree of success in limited clinical studies. Both, however, will require further evaluation and proof of clinical applicability. One recommends glass wool columns for semen filtration, while the other utilizes human serum albumin columns for the same purpose. The first one is discussed in another chapter, while the second will be described in the following pages.

2. THE TECHNIQUE OF SPERM SEPARATION ON ALBUMIN COLUMNS

The technique of sperm separation on albumin columns was described originally as a technique for isolation of Y-chromosome-bearing spermatozoa
(Ericsson et al. 1973). The authors observed that a leading semen fraction which
passed through several concentration gradients of bovine serum albumin (BSA)
was characterized by a high percentage of fluorescent Y-body(F-body)-bearing
spermatozoa and by high motility. About 85% of the spermatozoa in the separated semen sample contained F-body and 98% were motile. Both percentages
were significantly increased as compared to the original sample. Simultaneously,
a decrease in the percentage of abnormal forms and freedom of cellular debris
were observed in the isolated specimen. The isolation of Y-chromosome-bearing
spermatozoa was not consistent in subsequent studies with this technique (Ross
et al. 1975) and the percentage of F-bodies after separation, although increased,
was generally lower than originally reported. However, most investigators reported a significant increase in motility and decrease in the percentage of abnormal spermatozoa and seminal debris in the separated fraction.

In principle, the technique involves layering of washed sperm over serum
albumin in vertical columns and allowing the progressively motile spermatozoa
to swim into the albumin and downward through several discontinuous gradients. The degree of separation of spermatozoa on the basis of the rapidity of
their progressive movement depends on several variables critical to this technique. The principal factors include the number, volume and concentration of
albumin layers and the duration of the procedure. They determine the swimming
distance and time, and the handicap to spermatozoa created by the changing
viscosity and, as a result, they determine the completeness of separation. Variation in these indices may account for the variable percentage of Y-spermatozoa
isolated by different investigators. The isolation of motile spermatozoa from
non-motile elements has been less difficult and more readily reproduced.

For separation the semen should be obtained by masturbation, collected in
a clean container, allowed to liquefy, and processed within one hour of collection. A complete semen analysis is performed on an aliquot of the ejaculate.
The remainder of the semen is diluted with an equal volume of Tyrode's buffer
(pH 7.4) and centrifuged at 2800-3200 rpm (approximately $1300 \times g$) for 10-15
minutes. The supernatant is then decanted and the sperm pellet is resuspended
in Tyrode's buffer to give an approximate concentration of $20\text{-}60 \times 10^6$
spermatozoa/ml. The sperm suspension prepared in this manner is ready to be
layered in 0.5 ml aliquots on top of salt-poor human serum albumin (HSA)
columns. Isolation columns are made from 23-cm Pasteur pipettes heat-sealed
at the point of tapering.

To facilitate the maximum separation and simultaneously to achieve the
highest recovery of motile spermatozoa from a specific semen specimen, either

one or two-layer HSA columns are prepared. If sperm density and motility are essentially within the normal range, a two-layer HSA technique is recommended to remove abnormal and non-motile spermatozoa, as well as other cellular and non-cellular debris. For this purpose 1.0 ml of 7.5% HSA is layered in the columns over 0.5 ml of 17.5% HSA. This modification of the technique isolates a highly motile, clean semen fraction but permits the recovery of only a small proportion of motile spermatozoa from the original specimen (Figure 1).

Oligospermic specimens and especially those with significantly decreased motility should be processed according to the one-layer technique. The isolation columns contain only 1.0 ml of 7.5% or 10% HSA. The one-layer technique is used in place of the two-layer technique to increase the yield of motile spermatozoa. The separation is, however, less complete and some abnormal spermatozoa and some seminal debris may be found in the final isolated fraction (Figure 1).

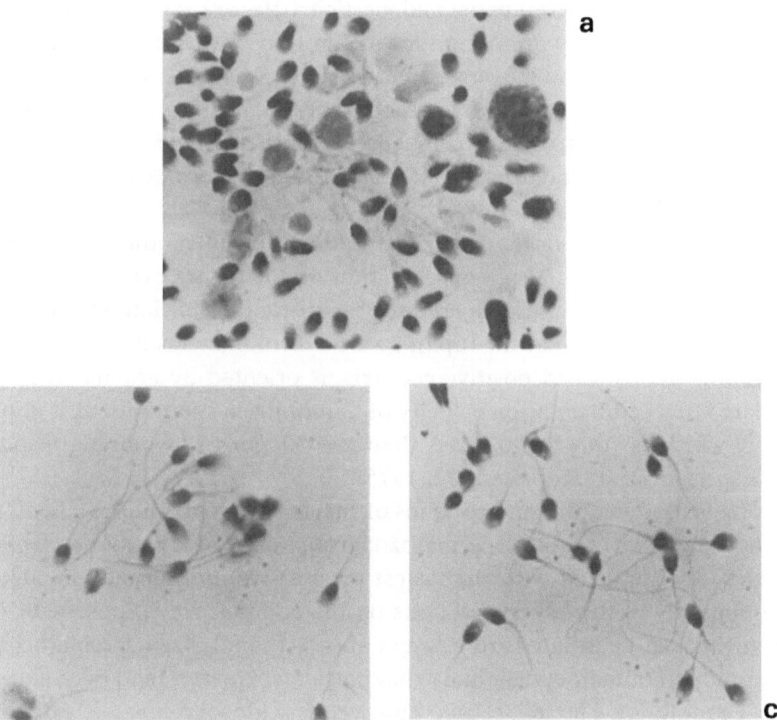

Figure 1. Photomicrograph of a semen specimen characterized by oligospermia, teratosermia and decreased motility (× 520): (a) prior to albumin filtration; (b) after filtration through 7.5% HSA; (c) after filtration through 7.5% and 17.5% HSA.

The number of isolation columns used for a given specimen is determined by the total number of spermatozoa in the ejaculate, with approximately $10\text{-}30 \times 10^6$ spermatozoa in 0.5 ml of Tyrode's buffer being layered on each column. The columns are kept in a vertical position at room temperature and at one hour the sperm suspension at the top of the column is removed. In the two-layer technique the 7.5% HSA is removed half an hour later. In the one-layer method the upper tenth of the 7.5% or 10% HSA is pipetted off with the sperm suspension. In both modifications of the technique it is the residual HSA at the bottom of the column which contains the most active spermatozoa. The bottom layers from all columns are collected, pooled and centrifuged at 2800-3200 rpm for 10-15 minutes. The supernatant is removed and the sperm pellet is re-suspended in 0.5-1.0 ml of Tyrode's buffer. This final sperm suspension is then used for AIH. Aliquots from the final specimen as well as from all specimens during the previous steps in the procedure are taken for semen analysis.

The velocity and orientation of spermatozoal movement in the albumin column are the result of interaction between complex and frequently opposing forces. Immobilized spermatozoa and inert particles are exposed to the effect of two main, diametrically opposing forces of gravity and viscosity. The resulting downward sedimentation movement and its velocity depend on the mass, size and shape of each particle and on the viscocity of the medium. Furthermore, inert particles experience a torque which depends on their shape and results in their tendency to a specific orientation (Roberts 1972). In case of spermatozoa, this orientation will be head downward.

The forces controlling the velocity and direction of motile spermatozoa in albumin columns of varying concentration gradients are even more complex. Suffice it to say that motile spermatozoa orient their swimming movements downward when placed at the top of a vertical column. Their active swimming downward, the so-called positive geotaxis, is oriented by gravity. It has been calculated that sedimentation velocity of immobilized spermatozoa is about 0.3 $\mu\text{m.s}^{-1}$, which is considerably less than the 50 $\mu\text{m.s}^{-1}$ swimming velocity of motile spermatozoa (Roberts 1972, 1975).

In practical terms, albumin columns of varying concentration gradients facilitate the separation of motile spermatozoa from non-motile forms and from inert particles. Spermatozoa with the fastest progressive motion may be identified predominantly in the lowest fractions on the column, while those with slower movements can be isolated from layers above. Immobilized spermatozoa, epithelial and inflammatory cells and other particulate matter tend to remain at the top of the column. The separation, however, is seldom complete. The degree of completeness depends on the number of layers of HSA and their concentration.

Using the two-layer technique and semen sample with close to normal sperm concentration and motility it is readily feasible to isolate a fraction characterized by over 80% motility and less than 20% abnormal forms (Ericsson et al. 1973;

Dmowski et al. 1978b). This fraction will only contain, however, between 4 and 12% of the original motile sperm count. In infertile men, who have a low count of motile spermatozoa in initial specimens, this may mean recovery of less than 4×10^6 of motile spermatozoa in the isolation fraction (Dmowski et al. 1978a; Glass and Ericsson 1978). Although it has not been determined how many spermatozoa are needed in the AIH specimen to accomplish pregnancy, no conceptions occurred when numbers lower than 4 million were used (Dmowski et al. 1978b).

An increase in the recovery of motile spermatozoa from the albumin column can be achieved by: (1) exposing a larger number of spermatozoa directly to the albumin (increase in the albumin-sperm suspension interphase); (2) decreasing the number of albumin layers; (3) decrease in the height of the column; and (4) increase in the time of exposure. The first recommendation involves adjusting the sperm concentration in the suspension placed on each column. For specimens with low motility and a lot of debris this concentration should be closer to 20×10^6 spermatozoa/ml. It allows penetration of the albumin layer by a larger number of spermatozoa. The second and third recommendations result in a decrease of the total distance swum by spermatozoa, while the fourth permits slower swimmers and abnormal spermatozoa to catch up with the faster swimmers. Using these four methods either alone or in combination the recovery of motile spermatozoa may be increased to as high as 30% with a final fraction characterized by up to 74% motility and a 27×10^6 total sperm count (Glass and Ericsson 1978; Dmowski et al. 1978a).

Adoption of the above recommendations results, however, in a less complete separation. The final fraction, although cleaner than the original specimen, will contain abnormal forms, non-motile spermatozoa and seminal debris. The clinician may wish, however, to compromise on the quality of the final specimen in order to achieve an adequate quantity of spermatozoa and to increase the chance for success of the AIH.

The procedure of in vitro sperm separation using albuming columns may resemble to some extent the events taking place in vivo. Numerous investigators have suggested that the cervical mucus has the ability to filter selectively abnormal and non-motile spermatozoa, allowing only highly motile and morphologically normal sperm cells to arrive at the site of fertilization. This process could be one of the mechanisms preventing fertilization of the ovum by morphologically abnormal spermatozoa.

Selective filtration properties of the cervical mucus have been suggested by several in vitro studies. In one such study with capillary tubes filled with cervical mucus and placed in semen reservoirs, only motile and predominantly normal spermatozoa were found in the upper segment of the tubes (Perry et al. 1977). The filtering capacity of the cervical mucus appears to be equally efficient for various types of morphological anomalies. Only a small proportion (8-11%) of abnormal spermatozoa was found in upper segments of the capillaries, regardless of the percentage of abnormal spermatozoa in the semen reservoirs.

The concept of a filtering function of the cervical mucus receives further support from several in vivo studies in different species, evaluating motility and morphology of spermatozoa recovered from various levels in the female genital tract. One such study in women demonstrated progressive decrease in the percentage of immobile and abnormal spermatozoa when recovered from the vagina, uterine cervix, uterine cavity, and pouch of Douglas respectively (Hammerstein et al. 1977).

3. HUMAN IN VITRO STUDIES

Sperm separation on albumin columns has been studied by several investigators. The original report (Ericsson et al. 1973) claimed isolation of a highly motile semen fraction, high in Y-chromosome-bearing spermatozoa. After passage through three layers of bovine serum albumin (BSA) the initial sperm motility increased from 63 to 98% and concentration of Y-spermatozoa from 48 to 85%. Subsequent reports have not been in complete agreement as to the percentage of Y-spermatozoa in the isolated fraction, but it is generally agreed that an increase was observed (Table 1). The majority of investigators reported, however, a significant 'clean-up' effect of this procedure on the abnormal semen.

Table. 1. Isolation of Y-spermatozoa from human semen using albumin columns.

Investigator	Technique	Maximum percentage Y-spermatozoa
Ericsson et al. (1973)	3 layers BSA	85%
Soupart (1975)	3 layers BSA	80%
Broer et al. (1977)	3 layers BSA	78%
David et al. (1977)	3 layers BSA	71%
Dmowski et al. (1978b)	2 layers HSA	80%

A decrease in the percentage of abnormal and non-motile spermatozoa and absence of cellular and non-cellular debris were observed (Table 2). The total sperm count and motile sperm recovery in the isolated fractions were variable and depended on the number and concentration of serum albumin layers and on the original quality of semen specimens.

As indicated in Table 2, the average increase in sperm motility after filtration was about 33%, while morphologically abnormal spermatozoa decreased by about 23%. Although the total sperm count in the isolated fraction varied between 3 and 37 million, the motile sperm count was much lower and ranged between 1.3 and 27 million. The lowest recovery of motile spermatozoa was about 4%, while 30% was the highest.

Table 2. Sperm filtration on albumin columns: in vitro results.

Investigator	Technique		Original specimen (mean values)				Isolated fraction (mean values)				
	Albumin	Concentration gradients (%)	Total sperm count ($\times 10^6$)	Motile (%)	Abnormal forms (%)	Motile sperm count ($+10^6$)	Total sperm count ($\times 10^6$)	Motile (%)	Abnormal forms (%)	Motile sperm count ($\times 10^6$)	Motile sperm recovery (%)
Ericsson et al. (1973)	BSA	6, 10, 20	—	72	—	—	—	98	—	—	12
Ross et al. (1975)	BSA	6, 10	—	63	—	—	—	98	—	—	12
David et al. (1977)	BSA	10, 15, 25	—	57	—	—	—	80	—	—	1-5
Glaub et al. (1976)	BSA	10, 15, 25	—	60	—	—	—	95	—	—	16
Ericsson (1977)	BSA	7.5, 17.5	—	53	—	—	—	88	—	—	23
	BSA	6, 15	—	37	—	—	—	86	—	—	—
Carruthers (1978)	HSA	10	192	14	—	27	9	38	—	3.4	13
			44	18	—	8	3	42	—	1.3	16
Dmowski et al. (1978a)	HSA	7.5, 17.5	119	41	48	49	6.3	80	26	5.0	10
	HSA	7.5	203	45	46	91	37	74	25	27.5	30
Dmowski et al. (1978b)	HSA	10, 20	363	41	47	149	8	77	14	6.2	4
Glass and Ericsson (1978)	HSA	7.5, 17.5	124	41	—	51	8	85	—	6.8	13
	HSA	10	120	36	—	43	17	66	—	11.2	30

Usually the total sperm count, motile sperm count, and motile sperm recovery in the isolated fraction were the highest when the one-layer technique was used. The highest motility, on the other hand, was achieved with the two- and three-layer techniques.

4. ANIMAL STUDIES AND APPLICATION IN ANIMAL HUSBANDRY

The technique of sperm separation on albumin columns has been used for filtration of the semen prior to artificial insemination in several animal species. The purpose of these investigations was to evaluate the effect of separation on the conception rate and sex ratio at birth. The studies have been performed in rabbits, cattle, horses, sheep and swine (Illyes et al. 1977, 1978; Goodeaux and Kreider 1978; Faust et al. 1976). Various modifications of the original technique (Ericsson et al. 1973), primarily in regard to the number and concentration of BSA layers, were employed.

Generally, the effect of the procedure on animal semen was similar to that observed in human studies. There was a significant increase in the percentage of motile and morphologically normal spermatozoa in the isolation fraction and a decrease in seminal debris.

Normal conceptions, gestations and normal births were observed following insemination in all species studied. The preliminary data available on conception rate for separated semen does not indicate significant change as compared to the whole semen. No information has been published as yet on sex ratio at birth in animals inseminated with separated semen.

5. CLINICAL APPLICATION AND RESULTS

The technique of sperm separation on albumin columns has found clinical application in male sex preselection and male infertility. It may also be of a potential clinical use as a sperm filtration procedure (1) prior to intrauterine insemination in women with a cervical factor of infertility; (2) prior to freezing or after thawing of semen in semen banking; and (3) prior to AIH in women with habitual abortions. Clinical and experimental studies on male sex preselection with this technique are discussed elsewhere.

Application of albumin columns to sperm filtration in the treatment of male infertility has been prompted by several reports indicating isolation with this technique of a highly motile, clean fraction from the human semen. In vitro studies with oligospermic and teratospermic semen of low motility, performed by different investigators, confirmed the initial impression (Table 2). Subsequent experimental data indicated that in several animal species semen separated on the albumin columns is capable of normal ovum fertilization resulting in normal pregnancy. In humans, the first conceptions with semen isolated on albumin columns occurred in couples requesting male child preselection (Dmowski et al. 1978b). The pregnancies were normal and were followed by deliveries of normal infants.

Although the technique and its purpose is somewhat different when used for male sex preselection, the pregnancies achieved indicate that spermatozoa after separation on albumin columns retain normal fertilizing potential. The minimal motile sperm count in the AIH specimen resulting in conception was in the range of four million.

When applied to male infertility the technique of sperm separation on albumin columns had variable results (Table 3). In one study (Glass and Ericsson 1978) no conceptions occurred in 19 couples after 67 cycles of AIH with separated specimens. The separation was performed with either the one or two-layer technique and the average motile sperm count in the AIH specimens was 11.2 and 6.8 million respectively. In another report (Dmowski et al. 1978b) male infertility and request for male child preselection were the reasons for a total of 68 cycles of AIH in 17 couples. The semen was separated according to the two-layer technique (10% and 20% HSA) and the motile sperm count in the AIH specimen varied between 4 and 8 million. Three conceptions and normal pregnancies resulted.

The incidence of conception appears to be related to the motile sperm count in the AIH specimen and therefore to the original motile count and the effectiveness of the technique in terms of separation and recovery. Sperm separation on albumin columns was performed prior to the AIH in 27 couples with a male factor of infertility (Dmowski et al. 1978a). The two-layer technique (7.5% and 17.5% HSA) was used in 21 couples for a total of 94 cycles without resulting conception. The average motile sperm count used for AIH was 5 million. The one-layer technique (7.5% HSA) was used in 12 couples for a total of 22 AIH cycles resulting in four conceptions. The average motile sperm count used for insemination in this group was 27 million. In three patients who conceived the motile sperm count in the AIH specimen exceeded 10 million; it was just over 5 million in one. All pregnancies terminated in the delivery of healthy infants, two males and two females.

It is interesting to note that two of four patients who conceived as a result of AIH after semen separation with the one-layer technique had previously undergone AIH for several cycles with the sperm separated using to two-layer technique but without resulting conception. It appears from the above that the two-layer separation may produce a rather low number of motile spermatozoa, frequently too low for a successful AIH. The one-layer technique seems to be more useful in this respect. The usefulness of the one-layer technique in improving the chances of conception in couples with male factor infertility has

Table 3. Treatment of male infertility using sperm filtration on albumin columns and AIH

Investigator	Technique of:		Total number		Pregnancies	Motile sperm count ($\times 10^6$)		Contributory female factors
	Filtration	AIH	Patients	AIH cycles		Mean of AIH specimen	Lowest resulting in conception	
Glass and Ericsson (1978)	1 (2) layers	IU	19	67	0	11 (7)	—	yes
Dmowski et al. (1978a)	2 layers	IC + IU	21	68	0	5	—	yes
	1 layer	IC + IU	12	22	4	27	5	yes
Dmowski et al. (1978b)	2 layers	IC + IU	17	68	3	6	4	yes
Black and Servy (1978, personal communication)	1 layer	IC	12	50	4	9	8	no

IC: intracervical;
IU: intrauterine.

been observed also by other investigators (Black and Servy 1978, personal communication).

As demonstrated in Table 2 and Table 3 the recovery of motile spermatozoa was rather low in all studies, but expecially low when two or three-layer techniques were used. The relatively few conceptions achieved are probably related to the patient selection and the rather low count of motile spermatozoa used for AIH. The sperm filtration procedure was performed in all studies as a last-resort therapy after many years of infertility and following failure of other techniques. Furthermore, in all reported studies a significant contribution of female factors to the infertility was noted.

The technique of sperm filtration on albumin columns may be useful prior to intrauterine insemination. Such a clinical need may arise in women with the cervical factor of infertility not responding to other methods of treatment (Kremer et al. 1977; Insler et al. 1977). Filtration of the semen sample on albumin columns removes abnormal spermatozoa, epithelial cells, inflammatory cells and seminal debris. Furthermore, seminal plasma is also removed. Intrauterine insemination with the separated semen is, therefore, less likely to cause the inflammatory reaction or painful uterine contractions observed at times when whole semen is used for this purpose (Glass and Ericsson 1978; Carruthers 1978).

The high incidence of spontaneous abortion in couples with the male factor of infertility has been observed by several investigators and may be related to the high percentage of morphologically abnormal spermatozoa in their semen. Sperm filtration on albumin columns could potentially lower this incidence by isolating for insemination only spermatozoa with strong viability and structural normalcy. About 60% of first-trimester abortions are associated with chromosomal anomalies. It is possible that some of these conceptions occurred as a result of the ova being fertilized by spermatozoa abnormal in chromosomal composition. It is not known, but not unlikely, that morphologically abnormal spermatozoa may carry genetic anomalies.

Although the technique of sperm filtration on albumin columns has been shown to be effective in removing only morphologically abnormal spermatozoa it is possible that spermatozoa with abnormal chromosome composition and specifically those with additional chromosomes are also removed or retarded enough to be excluded from the final isolation fraction. The technique would be of considerable clinical value if it could exclude such spermatozoa and increase the probability of a normal conception. Unfortunately, there is no scientific data supporting this hypothesis. On the contrary, some studies (David et al. 1977) seem to suggest that spermatozoa with a specific type of chromosomal error may be found in higher concentrations in the isolated fraction of the semen. The authors have shown a statistically significant increase in the percentage of spermatozoa with two F-bodies and presumably with YY configuration after separation on albumin columns. Although it has been questioned whether spermatozoa with two F-bodies have indeed YY configuration or an incompletely condensed single Y-chromosome (Sumner and Robinson 1976), such a possibility should be kept in mind.

Another potential clinical application of sperm separation is in semen cryobanking. Filtration prior to or after freezing could increase the quality of the semen used for artificial donor insemination (AID). Some preliminary data seem to indicate that such procedure could be of a potential value at least in terms of sperm motility in the AID specimen (Glaub et al. 1976; Ericsson 1977). However, whether this effect could be correlated with the increase in conception rate following AID with freeze-preserved specimens remains to be proven.

REFERENCES

Amelar RD, Dubin L: A coital technique for the promotion of fertility. *Urology* 5:228, 1975.
Amelar RD, Hotchkiss RS: The split ejaculate: its use in the management of male infertility. *Fertil Steril* 16:46, 1965.
Broer KH, Dauber V, Kaiser R: The selection of Y-chromatin positive spermatozoa and subsequent in vitro penetration through cervical mucus. *Int J Fertil* 22:125, 1977.
Carruthers GB: Clinical experience with the separation of mobile spermatozoa for the treatment of oligospermia. Presented at the first international symposium on AIH and male subfertility, Bordeaux, 1978.
David G, Jeuling C, Boyce A, Schwartz D: Motility and percentage of Y- and YY-bearing spermatozoa in human semen samples after passage through bovine serum albumin. *J Reprod Fertil* 50:377, 1977.
Dmowski WP, Gaynor L, Lawrence M, Rao R, Scommegna A: Isolation of motile spermatozoa in oligospermic males prior to AIH of the wife. Presented to the first international symposium on AIH and male subfertility, Bordeaux, 1978a.
Dmowski WP, Gaynor L, Rao R, Lawrence M, Scommegna A: X and Y sperm separation and clinical experience with AIH separated for male sex preselection. Presented at the first international symposium on AIH and male subfertility, Bordeaux, 1978b.
Eliasson RJ: Standards for investigation of human semen. *Andrologia* 3-49, 1971.
Ericsson RJ, Langevin CN, Nishino M: Isolation of fractions rich in human Y sperm. *Nature* 246:421, 1973.
Ericsson RJ: Isolation and storage of progressively motile human sperm. *Andrologia* 9:111, 1977.
Faust AM, Kreider JL, Ericsson RJ, Goodeaux SD, Godke RA: Isolation of progressively motile spermatozoa from bull semen. *J Animal Science* 43:209, 1976.
Farris EJ, Murphy DP: The characteristics of the two parts of the partitioned ejaculate and the advantages of its use for intrauterine insemination. *Fertil Steril* 11:465, 1960.
Glass RH, Ericsson RJ: Intrauterine insemination of isolated motile sperm. *Fertil Steril* 29:535, 1978.
Glaub JC, Mills RN, Katz DF: Improved motility recovery of human spermatozoa after freeze preservation via a new approach. *Fertil Steril* 27:1283, 1976.
Goodeaux SD, Kreider JL: Motility and fertility of stallion spermatozoa isolated in bovine serum albumin. Presented at the annual meeting of the southern division of the American society of animal science, Houston, 1978.
Hammerstein J, Zielske F, Kratzsch E, Koch UJ: Sperm migration throughout the female genital tract in relation to the time of ovulation. In: *The uterine cervix in reproduction*, Insler V, Bettendorf G (eds), Stuttgart, Georg Thieme, 1977, p 238.
Illyes DR, Warren WR, Baham A, Kreider JL, Godke RA: Freezing separated bovine spermatozoa. *J Animal Science* 45:171, 1977.

Illyes DR, Warren WR, Baham A, Kreider JL, Godke RA: Effect of fructose supplementation on separated bovine spermatozoa. Abstract 817, Michigan state meetings of the American dairy science society, 1978.

Insler V, Bernstein D, Glezerman M: Diagnosis and classification of the cervical factor of infertility. In: *The uterine cervix in reproduction*, Insler V, Bettendorf G (eds), Stuttgart, Georg Thieme, 1977, p 253.

Kleegman SJ, Kaufman A: *Infertility in women*, Philadelphia, Davis, 1966.

Kremer J, Jager S, Slochteren-Draaisma T van: Treatment of infertility due to antisperm antibodies. In: *The uterine cervix in reproduction*, Insler V, Bettendorf G (eds), Stuttgart, Georg Thieme, 1977, p 249.

Perry G, Glezerman M, Insler V: Selective filtration of abnormal spermatozoa by the cervical mucus in vitro. In: *The uterine cervix in reproduction*, Insler V, Bettendorff G (eds), Stuttgart, Georg Thieme, 1977, p 118.

Roberts AM: Gravitational separation of X and Y spermatozoa. *Nature* 238:223, 1972.

Roberts AM: The biased random walk and the analysis of micro-organism movement. In: *Proceedings of the symposium on swimming and flying in nature*, vol 1, Wu TY, Brennan C, Brokaw CJ (eds), New York, Plenum, 1975.

Ross A, Robinson JA, Evans HJ: Failure to confirm separation of X- and Y-bearing human sperm using BSA gradient. *Nature* 253:354, 1975.

Soupart P: MGA-M appearance in ejaculated human sperm. *Proc Soc Study Reprod* 8:120, 1975.

Speroff L, Glass RH, Kase NG: *Clinical gynecologic endocrinology and infertility*, Baltimore, Williams and Wilkins, 1978 (2nd ed).

Sumner AT, Robinson JA: A difference in dry mass between the heads of X- and Y-bearing human spermatozoa. *J Reprod Fertil* 48:9, 1976.

Syner FN, Moghissi KS, Yanez J: Isolation of a factor from normal human semen that accelerates dissolution of abnormally liquefying semen. *Fertil Stèril* 26:1064, 1975.

Tyler ET: *Sterility*, New York, McGraw-Hill, 1961.

9. SEPARATION OF X AND Y SPERMATOZOA FOR SEX PRESELECTION

R.J. ERICSSON, W.P. DMOWSKI, K.H. BROER and G. GASSER

1. SEX CHROMOSOMES AND THE MALE GAMETE

The heterogametic sex (X or Y chromosome) is male in mammals, female in birds and in those reptiles examined so far, while in fish and amphibia both systems are found (Mittwoch 1971). Sex chromosome differences between the sexes are the presence or absence of a Y chromosome and the number of X chromosomes. An interesting theory states that different chromosome constitutions have a direct effect on rates of cell proliferation (Mittwoch 1970). Embryonically this theory applies to gonadal development; the gonadal rudiment is bipotential until the rate of growth at a certain stage of development influences its outcome. If a Y chromosome is present the dominant gonad develops (testis in mammals and ovary in birds). In the absence of a Y chromosome, the less dominant gonad develops in the homogametic sex. The cell proliferation theory is not, however, entirely adequate to explain the larger size of men and the superiority in number of gametes. What really sets aside men from women is their heterogametic nature.

The human Y chromosome does associate with the X chromosome; it does so during meiosis. Whether the chromosomes form a true chiasma is uncertain but an association is known for the short arm of the Y chromosome with the X chromosome during first meiotic prophase (Pearson and Bobrow 1970a). It is possible, with electron microscopy, to follow human pachytene X and Y chromosomes from partial synapsis through precocious disjunction and end-to-end attachment (Moses et al. 1975). Mitosis and meiosis are thought to be well-controlled events and seemingly free of gross errors; unfortunately this view is not supported by experimental data on the Y chromosome. Robinson and Buckton (1971) have established in man, at interphase and mitosis, eight abnormalities of the Y chromosome. The frequency of meiotic errors involving the Y chromosome of normal human spermatozoa is about 2.5% (Pawlowitzki and Pearson 1972). It is possible that the same frequency of aneuploidy in all chromosomes would result in 38% of gametes abnormal. Normalcy, location and identification of sex chromosomes in the male gamete is more complex than originally thought (not a new insight in biological theory).

This chapter is devoted primarily to cytogenetics of human X and Y spermatozoa, to include separation of gametes based on (1) sex chromosome, (2) viability, and (3) normalcy. All separations require manipulation of sperm in one manner or another.

2. RESEARCH IN SPERM CYTOGENETICS

The ability to stain and identify the Y chromosome in cells of the human male has furthered research in sperm cytogenetics more than any other recent technique or concept (Zech 1969; Pearson and Bobrow 1970b). It is now established that the Y body (fluorescent dot) seen in human sperm, stained with a fluorochrome, is part of the Y chromosome (Barlow and Vosa 1970). Others used the technique to explore different facets of sperm cytogenetics: Sumner et al. (1971) and later Pearson et al. (1973) began by confirming the theoretical value of 4% less DNA in Y sperm than in X sperm. Research is not limited to the Y chromosome; other chromosomes and other stains are under intense investigation due, in part, to the success of Y-sperm identification (Pearson 1972).

The phenotype of spermatozoa in relation to genetic content is a logical way to approach differences in the two sperm types (Beatty 1971). One established theory is that X and Y spermatozoa are not physically identical, since X and Y chromosomes differ greatly in size. Beatty (1971) believes the difference may be slight; Roberts (1972) is more specific for human sperm, saying the two types have a 1% difference in head radius. Pearson et al. (1973) have evidence for a 7% larger surface area of human X sperm compared to Y sperm. They go on to say, depending upon the assumptions made regarding the thickness of the sperm head, that this difference, when expressed in terms of volume, is increased by one or two orders of magnitude. The extra DNA in the X sperm cannot explain the large volume difference and therefore the question is raised as to whether some form of haploid expression is operative. Human sperm differences, based on the mass of all chromosomes, have been calculated such that 85.7% of the Y-bearing sperm can be expected to be lighter than all X-bearing sperm, and 99.2% would be lighter than all but 0.006% of the X-bearing sperm (Bahr 1971).

The truly or mathematically computed lighter Y sperm is used to advance the theory of sex ratio at birth based on preferential progress of Y sperm through the female reproductive tract (Roberts 1972). The swimming velocity of Y sperm is only 0.15% greater when calculated on the lesser amount of DNA, but it seems unlikely from the preceding discussion that DNA is the only difference between the two sperm types (Roberts 1972). Spermatozoa orient their swimming movements downward when placed at the top of a vertical column; Roberts (1975) gives the swimming rate in a dextran column at around 10 μm.s^{-1}. This rate is considerably greater than the sedimentation velocity of immobilized sperm (0.3 μm.s^{-1}). The two forces acting on the downward swimming rate are gravity and viscosity. Without going into mathematical formulas and biophysics, suffice it to say that sperm movement in model systems is a complex phenomenon (Roberts 1975). If present cytogenetic theory holds then the size difference between the two sperm types can explain the results of Rohde et al. (1973), Ericsson et al. (1973), Goodall and Roberts (1976), David et al. (1977) and Broer et al. (1977), where Y sperm outdistance X sperm. Other model systems and experimental procedures are certain to be set up to exploit further the known and imagined differences between X and Y spermatozoa. Some known differences are listed in Table 1.

Table 1. Known and theoretical differences between human X and Y spermatozoa.

Difference	Explanation	Reference
DNA	less in Y sperm	Sumner et al. (1971)
Size	X sperm larger	Pearson et al. (1973)
Phenogenetics	X and Y genotypes	Beatty (1975)
Motility	Y sperm swim faster	Roberts (1972)
Identity	Y sperm positively recognized	Barlow and Vosa (1970)
H-Y antigen	More antigen on surface of Y sperm	Wachtel (1977)

Between 60 and 70% of all human conceptions (extrapolated as compared to recognized anomalies) are chromosomally abnormal, and this leads to a uniquely high rate of fetal wastage (Pearson et al. 1973). Considerable clinical benefit is forthcoming if human semen can be rapidly screened for genetic normalcy. Genetically abnormal sperm can only be separated out, under present conditions, by some physical means. This need to associate genetics with sperm morphology becomes more important as technology advances to identify sperm with chromosomal errors. The clinician needs methods capable of decreasing the probability of a genetically abnormal fetus. XYY males can now be screened, but no practical way is at hand to remove sperm bearing double Y chromosomes (Hulten and Pearson 1971; David et al. 1977). The most likely connection between sperm with chromosomal errors and genetically normal sperm is viability and morphological normalcy (a somewhat subjective measurement). In isolating sperm with strong viability and structural normalcy it may be that a high percentage of genetically abnormal sperm remain outside these parameters. Man is also unique in having semen with extremely high percentages of morphologically abnormal sperm, as compared to other mammals. Stress, diet, environment and personal habits may all join to create the anomalies of human semen.

3. CONCEPTS IN SEPARATING X AND Y SPERMATOZOA

3.1. Man

Shettles (1960, 1964, 1973) is credited with having had a major influence on sex preselection research in man. His work is controversial as he stresses concepts difficult to confirm or deny. For example, it is claimed that sperm bearing the Y chromosome have morphological characteristics distinct from sperm bearing the X chromosome (Shettles 1964), namely, that Y sperm are smaller, more round-headed, in contrast to larger, elongate-headed X sperm. He further states that the human testis may well be a mosaic in regard to production of X and Y spermatozoa. If true, the 1:1 separation of sex chromosomes, as part of the meiotic process during spermatogenesis, would be invalidated. Others, using a fluorometric stain to identify the Y chromosome, have recorded counts in human sperm approaching the theoretical ratio of X to Y spermatozoa (Barlow and Vosa 1970; Sumner et al. 1971; Ericsson et al. 1973; Schwinger et al. 1976). These latter data are in conflict with Shettles's statement, but proof of either concept must await sexing of offspring conceived from sperm selected for certain criteria.

Human semen holds greater promise for sex-preselected spermatozoa than do other mammalian species. The reason, of course, is the technological advancement whereby a fluorochrome identifies Y sperm (Zech 1969; Barlow and Vosa 1970). This new technology speeds up research processes manifold, since prior to this technique all experiments on sex-preselected spermatozoa gathered data by sexing fetuses or neonates (not the type of research normally done in man). Even now, other species, with the exception of the gorilla and vole, require sexing of concepti as a determinate of success or failure in sex preselection experiments (Pearson et al. 1971; Tates et al. 1975). Man is therefore in a unique position to be the recipient of expanded research devoted to isolating X and Y spermatozoa (Ericsson 1973; Glass 1977). It is almost inconceivable to use human patients for initial sex preselection experiments due to the limited number of willing participants, the length of the gestation period, and the lack of control over natural inseminations. Nonetheless, mankind may be the first mammalian species with a reliable, reputable method available for universal application. Again, confirmation over a period of time, through sex of offspring, is the ultimate truth. Shettles's method is available and receives clinical use, but insemination in relationship to ovulation is a haphazard thing and not too reliable for statistical analysis. Shettles's concept, now that Y sperm are identifiable, could be tested to learn if respective sex chromosomes do reside in sperm with characteristic morphological shapes. Whether the concept is proven or disproven is not as important as the idea behind it. Persistence in researching sex preselection is required, since resultant date are not easily accepted by the scientific and medical community.

Ericsson et al. (1973) base their results on indirect evidence – indirect because the sex of offspring from preselected sperm was not the end-point. They used the Y body, the distal end of the long arm of the Y chromosome, showing up as a bright fluorescent dot (Pearson 1972), as a means of measuring potential changes in X and Y sperm ratios. This may be an opportune way to gather data, but it is nonetheless indirect. This process merits our attention as it asks us to change our thought patterns on sperm density and sperm separation completely. One established method (under different guises) is to suspend spermatozoa in an acceptable medium, immobilize them (normally lowering ambient temperature), and allow the heavier X sperm (under gravity) to settle to the bottom of the column. Sumner et al. (1971) confirm that X sperm have more DNA. But the problem with the 'heavier' aspect is to what the greater weight is due – it may be biological variability, more DNA, presence or absence of acrosome, or some unknown reason. To break with tradition is to ignore heaviness and to look at sperm as a force within for active isolation. Ericsson et al. (1973) did so by subjecting human

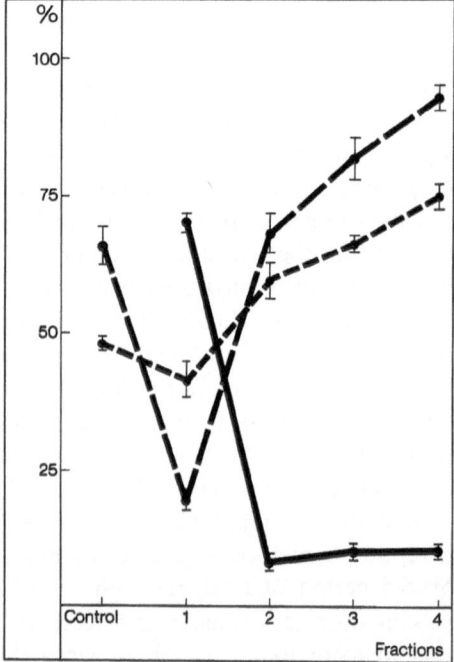

Figure 1. Human sperm layered over a column of 6 and 15% BSA. Fraction 1 is the original sperm layer; fractions 2 and 3 are upper and lower halves of 6% BSA; fraction 4 is 15% BSA. Long broken line, percentage sperm motility; short broken line, percentage Y sperm; solid line, percentage sperm recovery. Each point represents the mean ± SE of 9 experiments with 5 different donors. Note: two similar experiments where ovalbumin replaced BSA gave comparable results. Data from Ericsson et al. (1973).

sperm to situations designed to tax their swimming ability.

Figure 1 and Figure 2 give percentage data on sperm motility, sperm yield and Y sperm for the various fractions of isolation columns. The principle of Y-sperm isolation, as given here, is based on swimming sperm in a system that enhances differences in forward progression. Y sperm outswim X sperm under the handi-cap of swimming in a viscous medium. Time, distance and yield are crucial to success; if one is miscalculated, success is in jeopardy. For instance Ross et al. (1975) failed in five of six semen donors because of all the motile sperm taking part in the isolation process; the sixth donor produced added Y sperm in an isolation fraction and in this case sufficient numbers of motile sperm remained in the original fraction. Others have, however, rapeatedly isolated fractions with 70-80% Y sperm (Soupart 1975; Broer et al. 1977; David et al. 1977; Dmowski et al. 1979). The latter works confirm the method to be repeatable and reliable. Figure 3 is an example of human sperm prepared for Y-body identification. Under conditions such as this, Y bodies greatly in excess of fifty percent are counted (seven of the nine sperm present are scored as positive Y sperm).

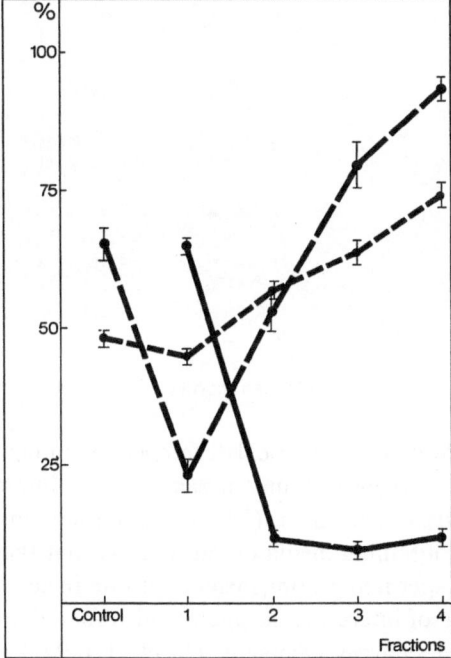

Figure 2. Human sperm layered over a column of 10, 15 and 25% BSA. Fraction 1 is the original sperm layer; Fraction 2 is 10% BSA; fraction 3 is 15% BSA; Fraction 4 is 25% BSA. Long broken line, percentage sperm motility; short broken line, percentage Y sperm; solid line, percentage sperm recovery. Each point represents the mean ± SE of 13 experiments with 5 different donors. Data from Ericsson et al. (1973).

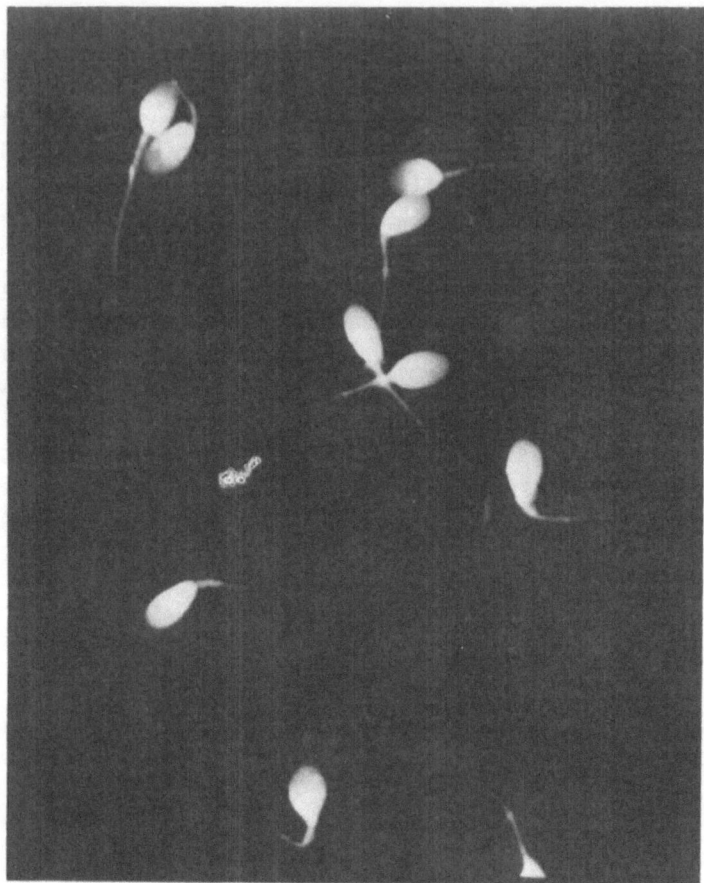

Figure 3. Fluorescent photomicrograph of human sperm (100×), fraction 3, Figure 1.

Apart from the known and theoretical differences in human X and Y spermatozoa listed in Table 1, there are three areas of active interest but of unconfirmed differences. Diasio and Glass (1971) allowed human sperm to migrate into capillary tubes containing media of varying pH, but their findings do not support the idea of Y sperm migrating faster or slower in acidic or basic cervical mucus. A further area of interest is the age-old idea that X and Y spermatozoa carry different surface charges. Yanagimachi et al. (1972) give chemical and morphological evidence for the entire surface area of human sperm to be strongly negatively charged, but this information did not prevent Lang (1973) from believing his ion-exchange resin technique to be capable of separating human sperm into X and Y fractions. Insemination of some 20,000 cows with sperm subjected to the ion-exchange resin system did not, however, significantly

Table 2. Percentage of Y-bodies in human sperm after centrifugation at 3000 rpm for 10 minutes.

N	Control	Centrifuged sample		
		supernate		
		High	Low	Sediment
1	48.7	42.3	45.5	47.6
2	49.7	51.2	48.8	46.7
3	47.5	52.6	47.6	47.2
4	49.1	37.5	39.5	46.4
5	48.8	44.1	40.8	47.3
6	50.5	42.3	46.8	48.8
7	47.0	45.2	47.1	47.0
8	45.8	51.6	45.6	47.2
9	45.6	37.4	37.2	47.6
10	43.2	40.5	36.9	42.6
$\bar{x}$	47.6	44.5	43.6	46.8
SD	±2.2	±5.6	±4.5	±1.6
t-test		no significant difference		

alter sex ratios in either direction. Centrifugation of fresh liquefied semen at 1500 rpm (327 g) to 3000 rpm (1307 g) for 10 minutes also did not change the percentage of Y sperm (Table 2) in the various fractions (Gasser et al. 1978).

3.2. Other species

Beatty (1974) compiled a bibliography on separation of X and Y spermatozoa; of these 106 references less than 10 percent dealt directly with human semen. It is more pragmatic, for example, to gather clinical data in cattle than in people. Thousands of offspring are obtainable within a year from cows artificially inseminated with sex-preselected sperm. Failure is less traumatic when it occurs in livestock and, more importantly, greater numbers make outcome less dependent on chance.

Attempts at separation of mammalian X and Y spermatozoa span many concepts but relatively few species (Table 3). Two ideas intriguing to a lot of researchers are that density and surface charge differ between the two sperm types. Research ideas less intensely investigated are froth flotation, antigen-antibody reaction, selected enzyme difference, pH and directed migration, and treatment of semen with hormones. References cited in Table 3 are not necessarily positive findings; sometimes they combine the original work or significant work on a selected method with findings either in support or denial of the method. No one concept has emerged as the most likely approach to practical separation of spermatozoa with regard to sex chromosome content.

Three divergent approaches, however, hold some short-term hope for sex

Table 3. Methods used to attempt separation of X and Y spermatozoa.

Method	Species	Reference
Electrical charge	Rabbit, man	Gordon (1957), Shishito et al. (1975)
Centrifugation	Bull, man	Lindahl (1958), Gasser et al. (1978)
Sedimentation	Rabbit, bull	Bhattacharya (1958), Schilling (1966)
Froth flotation	Rabbit	More O'Ferrall et al. (1968)
Sephadex gel filtration	Man	Steeno et al. (1975)
Enzyme content	Rabbit	Stambaugh and Buckley (1971)
pH	Man	Diasio and Glass (1971)
Immunology	Mouse	Bennett and Boyse (1973)
Sperm motility	Man	Ericsson et al. (1973)
Millipore filtration	Man	Shettles (1976)

preselection. These can be broadly characterized as density, enzymology, and immunology. Bhattacharya et al. (1966) could not repeat the earlier work of Bhattacharya (1958) on sedimentation, and therefore sex predetermination, of bull sperm. This inconsistency is a drawback to the method even though Schilling (1971) can repeatedly obtain positive changes in sex ratio up to 60% or 70% for either sex. To ignore sedimentation and centrifugation (sperm density differences) is to eliminate the majority of research done on sex preselection. It is argued that biological variability in density is greater among all sperm cells than is variability between the two sperm types, but since some successes are on record it would be premature to eliminate sperm density differences as a realistic approach to the problem, particularly if combined with another method. Enzyme content difference (Table 3) is a fairly recent and novel concept and can be viewed as another way to separate the two sperm types. Sedimentation is the vehicle to further nonequilibrium between an isozyme of LDH (characteristic of Y sperm) and absence of this isozyme (which X sperm are thought not to contain). Another creative idea is to make an H-Y antibody to combat the H-Y antigen, thus impairing fertility of sperm containing the Y chromosome. Bennett and Boyse (1973) tested this hypothesis in mice and were able to alter sex ratio 8% in favor of female progeny. One negative finding deserves mention because it helps in our understanding of spermatozoa and in the interpretation of some positive findings. For the purpose of sex control More O'Ferrall et al. (1968) used a method to float or sink rabbit sperm based on prior use of froth flotation to separate minerals (surface differences) and micro-organisms. The method failed.

4. SEX PRESELECTION IN THE CLINIC

Two approaches come to mind regarding how to test sex-preselected spermatozoa in the clinic. One is to do it the traditional way by artificially inseminating those women who seek out sex-predetermined offspring; the other approach is to gather data indirectly through couples seeking help for male infertility problems. The first method is more direct and therefore more objective in its aims, but it is also more prone to problems if the experimental procedure is not confirmed in the clinic. It is doubtful if any procedure used within the next decade, or ever, will be 100% reliable. Any method accurate 75-80% of the time will find users, even when they are made aware of the probability factor, but people currently seeking a sex-determined child tend to be motivated to conceive only if a child of the desired sex is assured. A child of the wrong sex or a child with congenital malformations would put most couples in a state of disillusionment. The state of the art is such that concerned scientists and practitioners view sex preselection claims with skepticism. Over-expectations can therefore be harmful, both to public acceptance and to personal lives. Even though couples may voice an open mind over their understanding of research procedures and final results in the clinic, they personally do not want to be recipients of any failures.

Childless couples with the male diagnosed as the probable subfertile partner are possible candidates for sex preselection in the clinic. These people are motivated to have a normal, healthy child; the sex of the resultant child is secondary to just having one. It could be explained to prospective patients that procedures used to improve semen quality may also change the ratio of Y to X spermatozoa, for example. Once they understood and accepted the possibility of a greater chance for male offspring, then inseminations could be undertaken. Admittedly, conception rates will be lower than from couples normal for fertility and interested in sex-determined children.

Sex preselection can be considered a form of genetic screening. Other areas of genetic screening are to select out, as much as possible, those sperm with chromosome abnormalities. It turns out that selecting for Y sperm also selects out spermatozoa of a more homogeneous order (Ericsson et al. 1973). These authors can 'clean up' semen to yield a population of spermatozoa almost entirely progressively motile and physically fit. Ross et al. (1975) confirm the isolation of motile and physically normal spermatozoa; they researched further and found up to 90% of original morphologically abnormal spermatozoa are selected out in the isolation process (see also Table 4). Whether these spermatozoa are in part genetically abnormal is not known directly, but it is not unlikely that some sperm contain both genetic and morphological anomalies. At first glance one wonders whether this in vitro approach is not just a less efficient method of duplicating what occurs naturally in cervical mucus. Perhaps this is true, but then again these procedures are for use by individuals who wish to predetermine the sex of a wanted child and must submit to artificial insemination.

Table 4 provides results from a clinical study with couples wanting a sex-preselected son (Dmowski et al. 1979). Semen from the men was processed using the modified procedures of Ericsson et al (1973). A fraction high in

Table 4. Sperm separation data in 37 couples requesting male child preselection using human serum albumin gradient columns (means ± SD).

| Couples | Before separation | | | | After separation | | | | | | | |
| | | | | | 10% HSA fraction | | | | 20% HSA fraction | | | |
	Total sperm count (× 10^6)	Motile (%)	Abnormal forms (%)	Y sperm (%)	Total sperm count (× 10^6)	Motile (%)	Abnormal forms (%)	Y sperm (%)	Total sperm count (× 10^6)	Motile (%)	Abnormal forms (%)	Y sperm (%)
Normal fertility n=20	510 (130-1243)*	45±13	37±11	46± 7	88±55	67±16	33±12	43± 4	16±10	83±9	17±11	71± 7
Subfertile n=17	363 (36-2218)*	41±19	74±16	45± 6	43±43	59±19	25±12	42±9	8± 6	77±15	14± 6	65±11
Pregnant n=10	395 (127-600)*	38±16	39±15	47± 4	65±54	64±17	29± 2	46±7	16±12	77±17	18± 2	69± 9

* range.

motile spermatozoa is obtained routinely, but what is not clear from Table 4 is that this fraction is also generally free of most round cells. The clinical goal is to take spermatozoa from the 20% human serum albumin (HSA) isolation fraction and use them for artificial inseminations. By inseminating into the cervical canal fewer viable sperm are necessary and since the procedure can readily be done under aseptic conditions, no problems should ensue. It is empirically thought that live normal sperm freed from dead sperm, abnormal sperm, and detritus will be more successful in fertility than these same live normal sperm inseminated with their unwanted brethren and debris. The number of viable sperm unencumbered by unwanted cells is a more useful way of measuring probability of conception than is the total number of spermatozoa. Results from a limited number of conceptions show the ratio of male to female offspring to parallel the ratio of Y to X sperm in the final fraction used for insemination (Table 4).

REFERENCES

Bahr GF: Separation of X- and Y-bearing spermatozoa by gravity: a reconsideration. In: *Sex ratio at birth: prospects for control, 1970 symposium*, Kiddy CA, Hafs HD (eds), American Society for Animal Sciences 1971, p 28.
Barlow P, Vosa CG: The Y chromosome in human spermatozoa. *Nature* 226-961, 1970.
Beatty RA: Phenotype of spermatozoa in relation to genetic content. In: *Sex ratio at birth: prospects for control, 1970 symposium*, Kiddy CA, Hafs HD (eds), American Society for Animal Sciences, 1971, p 10.
Beatty RA: Bibliography on separation of X and Y spermatozoa. *Biblphy Reprod* 23:1, 1974.
Beatty RA: The phenogenetics of spermatozoa. In: The biology of the male gamete, Duckett JD, Racey PA (eds). *Biolog J Linnean Soc* 7 (suppl 1): 291, 1975.
Bennett D, Boyse EA: Sex ratio in progeny of mice inseminated with sperm treated with H-Y antiserum. *Nature* 246:308, 1973.
Bhattacharya BC: Sex control in mammals. *Z Tierzücht Züchtungsbiol* 72:250, 1958.
Bhattacharya BC, Bangham AD, Cro RJ, Keynes RD, Rowson LEA: An attempt to predetermine the sex of calves by artificial insemination with spermatozoa separated by sedimentation. *Nature* 211:863, 1966.
Broer KH, Dauber U, Kaiser R: The selection of Y-chromatin positive spermatozoa and subsequent in vitro penetration through cervical mucus. *Int J Fertil* 22:125, 1977.
David G, Jeulin C, Boyce A, Schwartz D: Motility and percentage of Y- and YY-bearing spermatozoa in human semen samples after passage through bovine serum albumin. *J Reprod Fertil* 50:377, 1977.
Diasio RB, Glass RH: Effects of pH on the migration of X and Y sperm. *Fertil Steril* 22:303, 1971.
Dmowski WP, Gaynor L, Rao R, Lawrence M, Scommegna A: Use of albumin gradients for X and Y sperm separation and clinical experience with male sex preselection. *Fertil Steril* 31:52, 1979.
Ericsson RJ: Conceptual contraception. In: Schering workscop on contraception: the masculine gender, Raspé G (ed). *Adv Biosciences* 10:299, 1973.
Ericsson RJ, Langevin CN, Nishino M: Isolation of fractions rich in human Y sperm. *Nature* 246:421, 1973.
Gasser G, Kaspar L, Mossig H: Attempts at separation of X and Y spermatozoa. Presented at the first international symposium on AIH and male subfertility, Bordeaux, 1978, p. 206.
Glass RH: Sex preselection. *Obstet Gynecol* 49:122, 1977.

Goodall H, Roberts AM: Differences in motility of human X- and Y-bearing spermatozoa. *J Reprod Fertil* 48:433, 1976.

Gordon MJ: Control of sex ratio in rabbits by electrophoresis of spermatozoa. *Proc Nat Acad Sci USA* 43:913, 1957.

Hulten M, Pearson PL: Fluorescent evidence for spermatocytes with two Y chromosomes in an XYY male. *Ann Hum Genet* 34:273, 1971.

Lang JL: Alteration of sex ratio at conception. *Chemtech* March:189, 1973.

Lindahl PE: Separation of bull spermatozoa carrying X- and Y-chromosomes by counter-streaming centrifugation. *Nature* 181:784, 1958.

Mittwoch U: How does the Y chromosome affect gonadal differentiation? *Phil Trans Royal Soc Lond* B259:113, 1970.

Mittwoch U: Sex determination in birds and mammals. *Nature* 231:432, 1971.

More O'Ferrall GJ, Meacham TN, Foreman WE: Attempts to separate rabbit spermatozoa by means of froth flotation and the sex ratio of offspring born. *J Reprod Fertil* 16:243, 1968.

Moses MJ, Counce SJ, Paulson DF: Synaptonemal complex complement of man in spreads of spermatocytes, with details of the sex chromosome pair. *Science* 187:363, 1975.

Pawlowitzki IH, Pearson PL: Chromosomal aneuploidy in human spermatozoa. *Humangenetik* 16:119, 1972.

Pearson P: The use of new staining techniques for human chromosome identification. *J Med Gen* 9:264, 1972.

Pearson PL, Bobrow M: Definitive evidence for the short arm of the Y chromosome associating with the X chromosome during meiosis in the human male. *Nature* 226:959, 1970a.

Pearson PL, Bobrow M: Fluorescent staining of the Y chromosome in meiotic stages of the human male. *J. Reprod Fertil* 22:177, 1970b.

Pearson PL, Bobrow M, Vosa CG, Barlow PW: Quinacrine fluorescence in mammalian chromosomes. *Nature* 231:326, 1971.

Pearson PL, Geraedts JPM, Pawlowitzki IH: Chromosomal studies on human male gametes. In: *Chromosomal errors in relation to reproductive failure*, Bove A, Thibault C (eds), Paris, Centre International de L'Enfance, 1973, p 219.

Roberts AM: Gravitational separation of X and Y spermatozoa. *Nature* 238:223, 1972.

Roberts AM: The biassed random walk and the analysis of micro-organism movement. In: *Proceedings of the symposium on swimming and flying in Nature*, vol 1, Wu TY, Brennan C, Brokaw CJ (eds) New York, Plenum, 1975.

Robinson JA, Buckton KE: Quinacrine fluorescence of variant and abnormal human Y chromosomes. *Chromosoma* 35:342, 1971.

Rohde W, Porstmann T, Dorner G: Migration of Y-bearing human spermatozoa in cervical mucus. *J Reprod Fertil* 33:167, 1973.

Ross A, Robinson JA, Evans HJ: Failure to confirm separation of X- and Y-bearing human sperm using BSA gradients. *Nature* 253:354, 1975.

Schilling E: Experiments in sedimentation and centrifugation of bull spermatozoa and the sex ratio of born calves. *J Reprod Fertil* 11:469, 1966.

Schilling E: Sedimentation as an approach to the problem of separating X- and Y-chromosome-bearing spermatozoa. In: *Sex ratio at birth: prospects for control, 1970 symposium*, Kiddy CA, Hafts HD (eds), American Society for Animal Sciences, 1971, p 76.

Schwinger E, Ites J, Korte B: Studies on frequency of Y chromatin in human sperm. *Hum Genet* 34:265, 1976.

Shettles LB: Nuclear morphology of human spermatozoa. *Nature* 186:648, 1960.

Shettles LB: The great preponderance of human males conceived. *Am J Obstet Gynecol* 89:130, 1964.

Shettles LB: Sperm morphology, cervical milieu, time of insemination and sex ratios. *Andrologia* 5:227, 1973.

Shettles LB: Separation of X and Y spermatozoa. *J Urol* 116:462, 1976.

Shishito S, Shirai M, Sasaki K: Galvanic separation of X- and Y-bearing human spermatozoa. *Int J Fertil* 20:13, 1975.

Soupart P: MGA-M appearance in ejaculated human sperm. *Proc Soc Study Reprod* 8:120, 1975.

Stambaugh R, Buckley J: Association of the lactic dehydrogenase X_4 isozyme with male-producing rabbit spermatozoa. *J Reprod Fertil* 25:275, 1971.

Steeno O, Adimoelja A, Steeno J: Separation of X- and Y-bearing human spermatozoa with the sephadex gel filtration method. *Andrologia* 7:95, 1975.

Sumner AT, Robinson JA, Evans HJ: Distinguishing between X, Y and YY-bearing human spermatozoa by fluorescence and DNA content. *Nat New Biol* 229:231, 1971.

Tates AD, Pearson PL, Geraedts JPM: Identification of X and Y spermatozoa in the northern vole, *Microtus oeconomus. J Reprod Fertil* 42:195, 1975.

Wachtel SS: H-Y antigen and the genetics of sex determination. *Science* 198:797, 1977.

Yanagimachi R, Noda YD, Fujimoto M, Nicolson GL: The distribution of negative surface charges on mammalian spermatozoa. *Am J Anat* 135:497, 1972.

Zech L: Investigation of metaphase chromosome with DNA-binding fluorochromes. *Exp Cell Res* 58:463, 1969.

10. THE SPLIT EJACULATE

J. COHEN, A. FARI, W.J. FINEGOLD, S. PROPPING and M.L. TAYMOR

Many couples are frustrated by infertility caused by deficiency in semen characteristics, e.g. oligozoospermia. This pathology has not been consistently corrected by medical therapy, but AIH using the split-ejaculate method has been offered as a reasonable alternative because of its simplicity and potential benefit. The distribution of spermatozoa in the semen of animals and man is not uniform throughout the entire ejaculatory process. A historical review of this phenomenon is shown in Table 1. By fractionating the seminal specimen during the ejaculatory process, one may use the more concentrated, better-quality portion in performing insemination in infertile patients. In man, the first part of the split ejaculate usually contains 76% of the total number of spermatozoa (MacLeod and Hotchkiss 1942). The ejaculatory process involves three events which occur

Table 1. Historical review of split ejaculate.

Author	Parameters studied
Hunter (1786)	Aspects of fractions of ejaculate
Broesike (1911)	Number of sperm in different fractions
Gutman and Gutman (1941)	Prostatic origin of acid phosphatases
MacLeod and Hotchkiss (1942)	Number and motility of sperm
Lundquist (1949)	Qualitative and quantitative study of different secretions
Mawson and Fischer (1953	Distribution of Zn in different fractions
Oettle (1954)	Interpretation of the interfraction differences
Harvey and Jackson (1955)	Application of AIH
Harvey (1956)	Mechanisms of ejaculation
Eliasson (1959)	Biochemistry of different fractions
Farris and Murphy (1960)	Application of AIH
Amelar and Hotchkiss (1965)	Application of AIH
Undholmer (1973)	Interpretation of the fraction differences
Fari et al (1976)	Localization of genital accessory glands infections

in a characteristic sequence (Amelar and Hotchkiss 1965). A scant secretion from the Cowper's glands initiates the ejaculation, is followed by the secretion from the prostate gland, the products from the testes, epididymes and the vasa deferentia. This is followed by secretion of the seminal vesicles. It is the first portion therefore of the ejaculate which normally contains the highest concen-

Table 2. Sequence of emission of the different secretions in the ejaculate.

Sequence of emission	% of total volume
1. Littre's and Cowper's glands secretion	insignificant
2. Prostatic secretion	40-45
3. Testis epididymis-deferens secretion (sperm)	5-10
4. Seminal vesicles secretion	45-50

tration of spermatozoa. This differential characteristic forms the basis for the use of the split ejaculate in AIH (Table 2). This phenomenon is true in about 80% of the cases. In 10%, the second portion contains the better quality and in the remaining 10% there is no difference.

1. PHYSIOLOGY OF EJACULATION

Ejaculation takes place during the third phase of sexual intercourse, which is divided into four stages: excitation, active phase, orgasm, and relaxation. At the end of the active phase contractions of the smooth muscles of the internal genital organs expel seminal fluid into the posterior urethra, where it is held. At the same time, the sphincter at the top of prostate contracts to inhibit the release of spermatozoa into the anterior urethra. The bulbo-urethral zone is filled, giving the man a feeling of an unavoidable event. Due to peristaltic contractions of perineal muscles, the secretions are transported into the urethra. Orgasm is characterized by a succession of rhythmic contractions at 4-5 seconds. Ejaculation takes place in a series of emissions, the first emission, from the vas deferens, being the richest in sperm count.

It is possible to divide at least two fractions of the ejaculate: the first containing the secretion of the prostate and the largest part of vas deferens; and the second

Table 3. Mean sperm concentration and chemical composition of first and second portions of human split ejaculate.

Semen characteristics	Fraction 1	Fraction 2
1. Mean volume (ml)	1.09	1.69
2. Percentage of total volume	39	61
3. Mean total count (millions)	270	88
4. Percentage of total no. of sperm	76	24
5. Mean motility	55% (grade 4)	38% (grade 2+)
6. Mean fructose concentration	157	377
7. Mean lactic acid concentration	71	48
8. Acid phosphatase (U/ml)	2760	300

Sources: Data from MacLeod and Hotchkiss (1942) and the literature.

containing the secretion of seminal vesicles and the remaining sperm (Table 3). However, only 80-90% of the patients follow this pattern; some 5-10% of the subjects have a richer second portion. This reversed pattern may occur without reversal in the sequence of emission of different secretions. Also this reversal may occur from time to time in patients usually responding to the common pattern. Certain neurologic drugs (amphetamines) may cause this induced pattern.

2. SEMEN CHARACTERISTICS IN SPLIT EJACULATE

In healthy men, the initial amount of the semen contains some 76% of all spermatozoa (MacLeod and Hotchkiss 1942). The motility of sperm in the first portion is unquestionably superior to the motility of those in the terminal portion. The high concentration of fructose in the second part implies that the seminal vesicles' secretions are released during the latter phase of the act. The lactic acid accumulates as an end product of the metabolism of the spermatozoa and is found in greater concentration in the portion of the ejaculate containing the denser concentration of sperm.

Amelar and Hotchkiss (1965) examined 522 semen specimens from 86 husbands. Sperm count was significantly higher in the first portion than in the second portion of the total specimen in 88% of the cases. In 5.8% of the cases, the two portions were similar, and in a further 5.8% of the cases sperm count in the second fraction was higher than in the first fraction. The viscosity of the whole specimen was normal in 61 cases and increased in 25 cases. In no case, of these 25 cases, was the viscosity greater in the first portion than in the second.

The motility was better in the first fraction than in the second or in the whole ejaculate in 57% and better in the first portion in 77%. Delafontaine et al (1976) studied the volume and concentration of the two parts of split ejaculate in three groups of 100 infertile husbands (Table 4). Fari (1969) studied split ejaculates from 260 husbands. The proportion of cases where the first fraction was more concentrated in sperm than the second fraction was only 69% when the total concentration of the whole ejaculate was less than 20 millions/ml. In 28-46% of the cases, the richest fraction of split ejaculate was less concentrated than the whole ejaculate. This fact is due to the day-to-day variations of sperm concentrations.

The higher fluidity of the first portion is due to proteolytic enzymes of the prostate; the better motility of this portion may be explained by the fact that the second fraction contains immature sperms or 'stale' sperms delayed in seminal vesicles and deferens ampullas since the previous ejaculation. It is also possible that motility is enhanced by prostatic secretion, but inhibited by seminal vesicle secretion.

Table 4. Mean volume and sperm concentration of first and second portions and total of human ejaculate in one hundred cases (Delafontaine et al. 1976).

Type	Fraction 1 volume (ml)	Fraction 2 volume (ml)	Total volume (ml)	Fraction 1 concentration (millions/ml)	Fraction 2 concentration (millions/ml)	Total concentration (millions/ml)
Normozoospermia						
53 cases	1,57	2,54	4,20	140	42	78
30-200 millions/ml						
Oligozoospermia						
38 cases	1,71	3,12	4,82	25	6	13
<30 millions/ml						
Polyzoospermia						
9 cases	1,61	1,72	3,39	588	80	266
>200 millions/ml						

3. THE USE OF SPLIT EJACULATE

During masturbation, the first several spurts of the ejaculate are collected in one vial whereas subsequent spurts are collected in another vial. AIH is then performed with the richest fraction of the ejaculate after verification in each case. When the couples are reluctant, or if it is inconvenient for them, to perform AIH, a special coital technique is advised. The husband withdraws his penis from the vagina after the release of the first portion of the ejaculate. The use of this technique is especially useful when the husband has a high semen volume.

4. INDICATIONS

The technique of AIH with the split ejaculate is indicated in the following cases:
1. Oligospermia with poor penetration of sperms in the cervical mucus;
2. Polyzoospermia (with the less rich fraction);
3. Asthenospermia when motility is less than 40% at the first hour;
4. Excess of volume of semen;
5. Hyperviscosity of semen.
In general, the technique is useful when the postcoital test is poor in spite of a good cervical mucus, even if sperm count is apparently good.

5. CONCEPTION RATE USING SPLIT EJACULATES

It is difficult to evaluate the success of different authors based in their reports because of the lack of international criteria, e.g. of the components of split

Table 5. Results from AIH utilizing the split ejaculate.

Author	Sperm count (millions)	No. cases	% pregnancies
Payne and Skeels (1954)	<20	27	15
Amelar and Hotchkiss (1965)	66% <40	39	56
Perez-Pelaez and Cohen (1965)	<40	38	26
Steiman and Taymor (1977)	20-40	7	29
	<20	22	23
Moghissi et al. (1977)	<50 or		
	<50% motile	60	22

ejaculate and the computation of the pregnancy rate. It is apparent, however, that pregnancy rate can be increased by AIH using the split ejaculate.

Amelar and Hotchkiss (1965) reported a 56% conception rate, but many of their patients had sperm concentrations greater than 40 million/ml. In those studies which adhered to more rigid requirements in terms of initial semen quality the conception rate was 25%. Table 5 shows the results from AIH utilizing the split ejaculate. In the series of Propping et al. (1978), 50 couples were inseminated, with a 12% pregnancy rate. The pregnancy rate was 20% when the infertile women were excluded. The pregnancy rate after intercourse reached 8% during the same observation period. Cohen (1979) performed some AIH 224 times on 73 couples with an average of three inseminations per couple. The

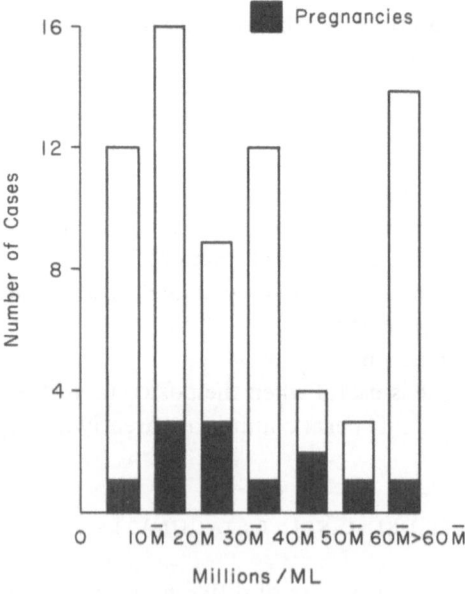

Figure 1. Distribution of cases according to concentration of sperms (millions/ml).

average pregnancy rates (13% for the total) were graphed with the distribution of sperm counts (Figure 1) and the distribution of sperm motility (Figure 2). Sperm motility does not seem to be related to pregnancy rate.

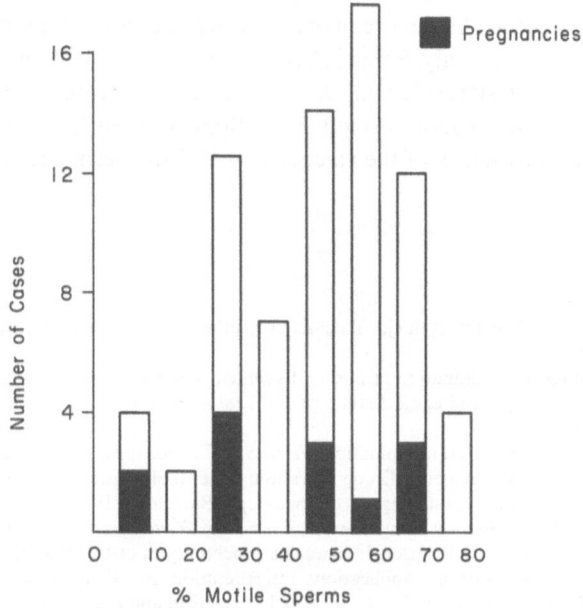

Figure 2. Distribution of cases according to motility (% motile sperms).

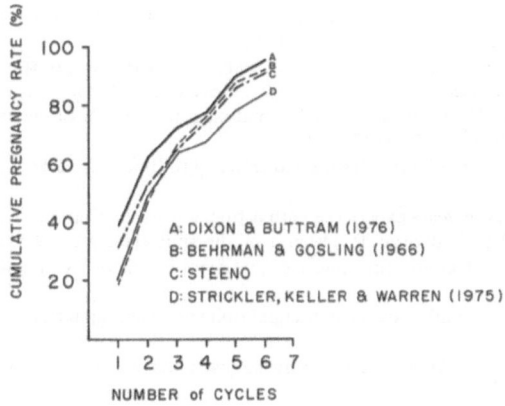

Figure 3. Insemination techniques.

6. CONCLUDING REMARKS

The technique of AIH with split ejaculate seems easy and efficient. It needs a minimum of material and may be accomplished by the doctor in his office or even by the couple at home. As the pregnancies occur after a small number of trials, couples accept the idea easily. Some 20% of pregnancies are obtained when other treatments have not succeeded in cases of (a) oligospermia with or without asthenospermia, and (b) poor postcoital test. Split ejaculate is actually the easiest way to improve the quality of the ejaculates with low sperm count.

REFERENCES

Amelar RD, Hotchkiss RS: The split ejaculate: its use in the management of male infertility. *Fertil Steril* 16:46, 1965.
Barwin BN: Intrauterine insemination of husband's semen. *J Reprod Fertil* 36:101, 1974.
Cohen J et al: Spermiologic and clinical study of artificial insemination with split ejaculate. *Fertil Steril* 28:310, 1977.
Cohen MR, Pandya G: Artificial insemination. *Fertil Steril* 5:430, 1954.
Delafontaine D, Cohen J, Grenier J: Étude spermiologique, biologique et chimique de l'éjaculat fractionné. Presented at the first congress of andrology, Barcelona, 1976.
Dixon RE: Artificial insemination using homologous semen. *Fertil Steril* 27:647, 1976.
Fari A, Verges J, Trevoux R, Belaisch J: Examens biochimiques et bactériologiques du plasma seminal humain I: méthodologie, applications, interprétation. *Rev Franç Gynéc* 71:663, 1976.
Fari A, Trevoux R, Verges J, Belaisch J: Cytologic, biochemical and bacteriologic study of human semen. *World Cong Fertil Steril* 9, 1977.
Finegold WJ: *Artificial insemination*, Springfield, Thomas, 1976 (2nd ed).
Guttmacher AF: Artificial insemination. *Ann NY Acad Sci* 97:623, 1962.
Hard AD: Artificial impregnation. *Med World* 27:163, 1909.
Harvey C, Jackson MH: A method of concentrating spermatozoa in human semen. *J Clin Path* 8:341, 1955.
Hill AM: Experience with artificial insemination. *Aust NZJ Obstet Gynaec* 10:112, 1970.
Home E: An account of the dissection of an hermaphrodite dog. *Phil Trans London* 89:157, 1799.
Langer G et al: Artificial insemination. *Int J Fertil* 14:232, 1969.
Lutwak-Mann C, Rowson LEA: The chemical composition of the pre-sperm fraction of bull ejaculate obtained by electrical stimulation. *J Agric Sci* 43:131, 1953.
MacLeod J, Hotchkiss RS: Distribution of spermatozoa and certain of chemical constituents in human ejaculate. *J Urol* 48:225, 1942.
McKenzie FF et al.: The reproductive organs and semen of the boar. *Res Bull Mo Agric Exp Sta* 279, 1938.
Nakamura MS et al: Seven years experience with artificial insemination. *Fertil Steril* 28:310, 1977.
Propping D, Tauber PF, Katzorke T: The use of the split ejaculate for homologous artificial insemination. Presented at the first international symposium on AIH and male subfertility, Bordeaux, 1978.
Sillo-Seidl G: The first child after artificial insemination with fractionated semen. *S. African Med J* 46:1517, 1972.
Speichinger J, Mattox JH: Homologous artificial insemination and oligospermia. *Fertil Steril* 27:135, 1976.
Steiman RP, Taymor ML: Artificial insemination homologous and its role in the management of infertility. *Fertil Steril* 28:146, 1977.

Taymor ML: The role of AIH in male subfertility. Presented at the first international symposium on AIH and male subfertility, Bordeaux, 1978.

Tyler ET: *Sterility*, New York, McGraw-Hill, 1961, p 340.

Ulstein M: Fertility of husbands at homologous artificial insemination. *Acta Obstet Gynecol Scand* 52:5, 1973.

White RM, Glass RH: Intrauterine insemination with husband's semen *Obstet Gynecol* 47:119, 1976.

11. ISOLATION OF MOTILE SPERMATOZOA IN OLIGOSPERMIC MALES PRIOR TO AIH

W.P. DMOWSKI, L. GAYNOR, M. LAWRENCE, R. RAO
and A. SCOMMEGNA

1. INTRODUCTION

The male factor is a significant cause of infertility in about 40-50% of childless couples. The severity of the problem is reflected in semen analysis which may indicate absolute sterility as in patients with azoospermia or a relatively minor problem as in patients with mild oligospermia. In the majority of infertile males morphologically normal, motile spermatozoa are intermixed in the semen with morphologically abnormal and non-motile forms, epithelial cells, pus cells, amorphous material, as well as with other cellular and non-cellular debris. It can be assumed therefore that separation of motile, morphologically normal spermatozoa from the abnormal forms and from sperm debris prior to homologous artificial insemination (AIH) should improve chances of conception in such cases.

Indeed, numerous reports have been published describing a variety of techniques for sperm separation prior to AIH and claiming varying rates of success in terms of improvement in semen quality and in facilitation of conception. Most of these techniques, however, have not been widely accepted, primarily because of little or no reproducibility of the results. A natural form of sperm separation through collection of different fractions of the ejaculate, so-called split ejaculate, is simple and has been widely used in clinical practice with reasonably good results. With this method seminal plasma is separated more or less efficiently from the sperm. Considered of value specifically in patients with inflammatory processes in the accessory sex organs, this technique makes available a concentrated semen specimen, relatively free from seminal plasma, for AIH. There is however no change in the percentage of abnormal or non-motile sperms and little change in the amount of sperm debris.

The technic of sperm separation reported by Ericsson et al. (1973) allows for isolation of progressively motile from non-motile sperm and from seminal debris. These results have been subsequently confirmed in this respect by Ross et al. (1975), Glaub et al. (1976), and Ericsson (1977). Most reports claim isolation of a clean semen fraction free of debris and containing up to 90% motile sperm with good forward progression. Encouraged by these reports and by the results of our preliminary studies with semen of normal males we performed, prior to the AIH, sperm separation using two modifications of Ericsson's technique in 25 couples with male factor infertility.

2. MATERIALS AND METHODS

The subjects in the study were 25 couples with a significant male factor of infertility as evidenced by oligospermia and/or low motility as well as a high percentage of abnormal forms in repeated semen analysis specimens. The characteristics of these patients are listed in Table 1.

All couples had been treated previously with various regimens including AIH with split semen specimens. In four of 25 couples no female causes of infertility were identifiable while in the remaining 21 various infertility factors were present in the wife. Ovulatory dysfunction in the form of anovulation or sporadic ovulation was observed in 17 wives; a relative tubal factor in the form of tubal phimosis or peritubal adhesions but with hysterosalpingographic evidence of tubal patency was observed in four; mild endometriosis in three; and short

Table 1. Characteristics of 25 couples undergoing sperm separation for male factor.

Average wife's age	31
Average husband's age	31
Average duration of marriage (yrs)	5.6
Average duration of infertility (yrs)	3.6
Couples with male factor alone	4
Couples with additional female factors	21
Anovulation	17
Relative tubal factor	4
Endometriosis	3
Short luteal phase	2

luteal phase in two. All wives with female factors contributory to infertility were treated simultaneously. Ovulation timing, utilizing basal body temperature (BBT) records, cervical mucus changes and vaginal cytology, was conducted during all cycles of insemination. Treatment with Clomid, HCG, or both, was used in patients with ovulatory dysfunction and short luteal phase. Hydropertubations were performed in patients with the relative tubal factor.

At the time of expected ovulation and after at least three or four days of sexual abstinence the husband was instructed to produce a semen sample by masturbation. Semen analysis as well as sperm separation procedure were then carried out as outlined below. Insemination (AIH) was performed with the separated semen specimen in a final volume ranging between 0.5 and 1 ml which was injected into the cervical canal at the level of the internal os. If ovulation was unpredictable,

AIH was repeated one to three times during the cycle until ovulatory response was noted. In some cases when ovulation occurred during the weekend when separation procedure was not performed the AIH was carried out with a split semen specimen.

2.1. Separation technique

The sperm separation procedure was performed as soon as liquefaction of the semen was complete; all manipulations were conducted at room temperature. Two modifications of Ericsson's technique were applied.

2.1.1. Two-layer technique.

Liquefied sample was diluted 1:1 with Tyrode's solution and then centrifuged at 3600 rpm for 15 minutes. The supernatant was discarded and the spermatozoa were resuspended in Tyrode's solution such as to contain approximately 60×10^6 of spermatozoa in each ml. Aliquots of 0.5 ml of sperm suspension were then layered onto isolation columns, the number of columns being determined by the total number of spermatozoa in a given sample. Each isolation column contained two discrete layers of human serum albumin (HSA). The lower layer consisted of 0.5 cc of 17.5% HSA while the upper layer consisted of 1 cc of 7.5% HSA. After one hour the top layer containing sperm suspension was removed and the remainder of the column was left for another 30 minutes. At that time 7.5% and 17.5% HSA layers were collected separately and centrifuged at 3600 rpm for 15 minutes. Supernatants were removed and spermatozoa were resuspended in Tyrode's solution. The sperm suspension obtained from the 17.5% HSA layer was used in a total volume ranging between 0.5 and 1 ml for insemination.

The total time between production of the semen sample and insemination was in the range of three to four hours. At each step in the procedure the total number of spermatozoa and the percentage of motile sperm were determined in the hemocytometer. The mean drive, that is, the speed of progressive motion across a distance of 0.05 mm, was measured with a stopwatch. The percentage of abnormal forms was determined subsequently on slides stained for spermatozoa. Also at each step in the procedure smears were prepared for fluorescent Y-body counts. The slides were air dried and fixed in 95% ethanol. Subsequently they were stained with quinacrine dihydrochloride and the percentage of Y sperm was determined by fluorescence microscopy.

2.1.2. One-layer technique.

This technique was essentially similar to the one described above with the exception that instead of two layers, one layer of 7.5% HSA was used in the column. All other steps in the procedure were identical. The sperm for insemination was recovered from the 7.5% HSA.

3. RESULTS

Total sperm count, sperm motility, percentage of abnormal forms, progressive drive, and percentage of Y sperms were the parameters evaluated at each step in the separation procedure. These data for the initial semen sample and for 7.5% and 17.5% HSA fractions are illustrated in Table 2. They are presented separately for one and two-layer techniques and are compared with similar data obtained for 18 normal males using 10% and 20% HSA separation (Dmowski et al. 1978).

The total sperm count and the percentage of motile sperm were lower in both oligospermic groups as compared to normal males, while the percentage of abnormal forms was higher and the forward progression of the sperm was more sluggish. There was a progressive increase in the percentage of motile spermatozoa in 7.5% and in 17.5% HSA fractions. Simultaneously, a decrease in the percentage of abnormal forms and an increase in the speed of forward progression was observed.

Both fractions, but specifically the 17.5% HSA fraction, were markedly freer of sperm debris, epithelial and pus cells and amorphous elements. A significant decrease in the total sperm count was observed in both fractions but specifically in the higher concentration of HSA. Motile sperm recovery was between 21 and 27% in the 7.5% HSA fraction and only 10% in the 17.5% HSA. The mean total count of motile sperm used for AIH in couples subjected to the two-layer technique was just over 4 million, while in those in whom the one-layer technique was used it was 16 million.

The analysis of clinical data is demonstrated in Table 3. A total of 121 AIH procedures with separated semen were performed in 83 cycles of 25 patients, resulting in four pregnancies and a pregnancy rate of 16%. There was one conception in four couples with male factor alone and three in 21 couples with both male and female factors. There were no pregnancies in the 19 couples in whom the two-layer technique was applied, all four conceptions occurring in the six couples in whom the one-layer technique was used.

Clinical information on four patients who conceived is presented in Table 4. Two conceptions occurred in the first cycle of AIH, one in the second, and one in the third. Three conceptions occurred in a cycle in which one AIH procedure was performed, while one patient conceived with three AIH procedures in a conception cycle. In two patients the AIH split procedure was performed in the conception cycle in addition to AIH separated.

The total count of motile sperm in the AIH specimen exceeded 10 million in three patients who conceived and was just over 5 million in one. All pregnancies were terminated in normal deliveries of healthy infants: two males and two females.

Table 2. Sperm separation procedure in 18 normal males and in 25 males with oligospermia.

| | Before separation | | | | | After separation | | | | | | | | | |
| | | | | | | 7.5% HSA fraction [a] | | | | | 17.5% HSA fraction [b] | | | | |
	Total sperm count ($\times 10^6$)	Motile (%)	Abnormal forms (%)	Drive (sec)	Y sperm (%)	Total sperm count ($\times 10^6$)	Motile (%)	Abnormal forms (%)	Drive (sec)	Y sperm (%)	Total sperm count ($\times 10^6$)	Motile (%)	Abnormal forms (%)	Drive (sec)	Y sperm (%)
Normal males, $n=18$, $\bar{x}$	258	59	29	1.12	48	59	75	24	1.09	50	20	86	13	0.92	70
Oligospermic males, two-layer technique, $n=19$, $\bar{x}$	124	42	48	1.26	48	19	59	41	1.16	49	5.5	78	27	0.96	51
Oligospermic males, one-layer technique, $n=6$, $\bar{x}$	170	35	58	1.25	—	24	68	29	1.03	—	—	—	—	—	—

a. 10% for normal males.
b. 20% for normal males.

Table 3. Analysis and results of AIH separated in 25 couples with male factor.

	No.	AIH cycles	Total AIH	Conceptions	Pregnancy rate (%)
Couples with male factor alone	4	9	11	1	25
Couples with additional female factors	21	74	110	3	14
Two-layer technique	19	68	97	0	0
One-layer technique	6	15	24	4	67
Total	25	83	121	4	16

4. DISCUSSION

The literature abounds with reports on numerous techniques designed to separate normal from abnormal spermatozoa in subfertile husbands prior to AIH of the wife. A variety of physical separation methods such as filtration, centrifugation, washing and pooling, and chromatographic separation have been reported with varying claims of success but generally with little or no reproducibility. Most of the techniques are rather complicated in use; their results have been erratic in hands of different investigators; and none has been generally accepted.

Our initial experience with Ericsson's technique as applied to normal semen specimens indicated a possible use for this procedure in isolation of a motile sperm fraction in subfertile males. Reports of other investigators on the effectiveness of this method in isolating a semen fraction free from debris and rich in highly motile sperm confirmed the original report of Ericsson et al. (1973) and have been in agreement with our experience. On Ericsson's recommendation we decided to use in the isolation columns two layers of HSA 7.5% and 17.5%, that is, concentrations somewhat lower than those used for Y-sperm separation. The selection of lower concentrations of HSA (7.5% and 17.5% versus 10% and 20%) was based on a presumption that spermatozoa of oligospermic males have less ability to move progressively through denser media than those of males with normal fertility.

As demonstrated in Table 2 our results indicate a significant increase in sperm motility and a decrease in the percentage of abnormal forms in the second HSA fraction. Simultaneously, an improvement in the speed of forward progression of the sperm was observed. However this improvement was accompanied by a significant decrease in total sperm count. It appeared that we were able to isolate only a small percentage of highly motile spermatozoa from the original samples. In view of the fact that the initial motile sperm count was low in our patients, we were not able to recover after separation with the two-layer technique adequate numbers of motile sperms to facilitate fertilization. This observation was confirmed by the fact that not a single conception occurred with 97 procedures performed in 68 cycles of 19 wives.

From analysis of sperm separation parameters in the lower concentration of HSA it became apparent that a significant proportion of motile spermatozoa was still present in that fraction at the completion of separation. We decided then to apply one-layer separation only, using 7.5% HSA concentration. With the one-layer technique a significantly higher number of motile spermatozoa could be isolated and the separated specimens were free of debris, had acceptable motility and a low percentage of abnormal forms. With the one-layer technique we were able to achieve four conceptions in six patients for a respectable 67% conception rate. Our observations regarding validity of a single-layer separation are in complete agreement with the data recently presented by Black et al. (1978).

Contrary to Ericsson's original report (1973) and our own data with 10% and 20% HSA concentrations used for sex preselection we were not able to detect any significant changes in the percentage of Y sperms before and after separation on 7.5% and 17.5% HSA columns.

In conclusion, the one-layer HSA separation technique, utilizing a 7.5% HSA concentration, can be used effectively to clean abnormal semen samples of non-motile forms, abnormal forms, other cellular and amorphous elements, and of sperm debris. It appears that this technique offers another chance for conception to a couple with male factor infertility. The two-layer technique does not appear to be of value in such cases, probably because of a significant drop in the total sperm count.

REFERENCES

Black JB, Peduto JC, Servy E: Male factor infertility treated by isolation of progressively motile sperm. Presented at the thirty-fourth annual meeting of the American fertility society, New Orleans, 30 March-1 April 1978.
Dmowski WP, Gaynor L, Lawrence M, Rao R, Scommegna A: X and Y sperm separation and clinical experience with AIH separated for male sex preselection. Presented at the first international symposium on AIH and male subfertility, Bordeaux, 1978.
Ericsson RJ: Isolation and storage of progressively motile human sperm. *Andrologia* 9 (1):111, 1977.
Ericsson RJ, Langevin CN, Nishino M: Isolation of fractions rich in human Y sperm. *Nature* 246:421, 1973.
Glaub JC, Mills RN Katz DF: Improved motility recovery of human spermatozoa after freeze preservation via a new approach. *Fertil Steril* 27:1283, 1976.
Ross A, Robinson JA, Evans HJ: Failure to confirm separation of X- and Y-bearing human sperm using BSA gradients. *Nature* 253:354, 1975.

12. RETROGRADE EJACULATION

B.N. Barwin, D. McKay, E.E. Jolly and A. Dempsey

1. introduction

Male factors, either absolute or relative, may be the cause of infertility in approximately 40% of childless couples. Retrograde ejaculation into the urinary bladder, a result of inadequate closure of the internal sphincter of the urethra, is an infrequent cause of male infertility. The incidence of retrograde ejaculation, however, may be expected to increase due to the higher incidence of vascular and colon surgery (Schirren and Hupe 1976), the increase in road accidents – transverse lesions (Kragt and Schellen 1978), as well as the increased use of drugs, particularly hypotensive drugs (Holister 1976; Kedia and Markland 1975).

Retrograde ejaculation is defined as the propulsion of seminal fluid from the posterior urethra into the bladder cavity, while the sensation of ejaculation is retained.

2. physiology of erection and ejaculation

Erection may be produced by sexual excitement, local stimulation of the glans penis, or as a sacral reflex arc (Potts 1957). It is controlled by the parasympathetic nerves or nervi erigentes (Retieff 1950). Parasympathetic activity produces vasodilation of the penile arteries and vasoconstriction of the penile veins resulting in engorgement of the cavernous bodies of the penis and urethra (Bol 1973). The pudendal nerve causes contraction of the bulbocavernosus and ischiocavernosus muscles. Also, skin sensory fibres of the penis are carried via the pudendal nerve and complete the arc. Although erection is essentially under parasympathetic control there may be an element of sympathetic control as 57% of patients who had removal of ganglia from levels as high as T1 and T2 had loss of power of erection (Andaloro and Dube 1975). Psychogenic factors play an important role (Kragt and Schellen 1978).

Ejaculatory control is a separate process and may be divided into three events. These are 'seminal emission', antegrade ejaculation, and bladder neck closure, and all are dependent on a reflex neural process (Kragt and Schellen 1978). Efferent impulses are sent from the genitalia via the pudendal nerve to the cerebral cortex. The efferent neural fibres travel through the anterolateral columns to the thoracolumbar sympathetic outflow and emerge through the T12 to L3 sympathetic ganglia. Branches from the hypogastric plexus innervate the epididymides and proximal portions of the vasa, whereas the distal portions of the vasa receive fibres from the vesical plexus, sympathetic and parasympathetic (Kimura et al. 1975). Therefore, the muscles of the epididymides, vasa, and prostate are mainly controlled by the sympathetic system. When these smooth muscles contract, sperm and seminal fluid are milked into the prostatic urethra, producing emission.

Once the seminal fluid is present in the posterior urethra several reflex actions occur. There is closure of the bladder neck, relaxation of the external sphincter with rhythmic contractions of the constrictor urethrae, bulbocavernosus and ischiocavernosus and also of other associated perineal muscles which propel the semen out via the urethra – 'ejaculatio propria' (Rieser 1961). Contraction of the bladder neck is under sympathetic control and prevents retrograde passage of semen. The external sphincter is relaxed by parasympathetic activity while the somatic nerves cause contractions of the striated muscles. Erection and seminal emission come about through a perfect combination of sympathetic and parasympathetic systems (Glezerman et al. 1976).

3. THE PATHOPHYSIOLOGY AND ETIOLOGY OF RETROGRADE EJACULATION

The mechanism responsible for the prevention of retrograde passage of semen is the closure of the bladder neck which is under sympathetic control (Glezerman et al. 1976). The receptor sites of this area have been shown to be of the α-type (Gennser et al. 1969). The stimulus for sympathetic activity of the bladder neck is the arrival of semen in the prostatic urethra. It follows therefore that any condition which inhibits closure of the bladder neck predisposes to retrograde ejaculation because semen can pass into the bladder more easily than through the urethra. The first stage of ejaculation is emission and takes place normally. The seminal fluid arrives into the prostatic urethra, but because of the failure of the bladder neck to claso retrograde, rather than antegrade, regurgitation takes place (Potts 1957). It is important to remember that an orgasm is achieved by these males (Hollister 1976).

4. ETIOLOGY

The causes of retrograde ejaculation may be divided into iatrogenic and non-iatrogenic (Ochsner et al. 1970).

4.1. Iatrogenic causes

There are two major iatrogenic causes. The first is incompetence of the bladder neck following surgical resection or repair for obstructive disease. Commonly incriminated in this respect is transurethral resection of the prostate gland, where Rieser (1961) found that 42% of cases subsequently developed retrograde ejaculation. Girgis et al. (1968) reported on eleven cases of retrograde ejaculation following surgery and demonstrated that the underlying cause was damage to the bladder neck. Using cystoscopy they found that the bladder neck was dilated, had no sphincteric action, and that the posterior urethra was visible to the verumontanum. Normally visualization does not go beyond the bladder neck because of the ionic contraction of the posterior sphincter. Similarly, Ochsner et al. (1970) reported that 33% of patients developed retrograde ejaculation following bladder neck revision either open or transurethral for obstruction.

The second iatrogenic cause results from interruption of the sympathetic innervation of the bladder neck with consequent failure of closure. Retrograde ejaculation has been reported in 10-64% of patients following bilateral lumbar sympathectomy (Leiter and Brendler 1967). Abdomino-perineal resection may also result in this condition, an incidence of 39% being found by Goligher (1951). Similarly, extensive retroperitoneal lymphadenectomy may damage the sympathetic nerve supply to the bladder neck resulting in regurgitant aspermia (Innes-Williams et al. 1950-1951). The aforementioned surgical procedures may also result in failure to ejaculate because of the interruption of sympathetic control of the muscles of the seminal vesicles, ampulla and ductus deferens, thereby preventing the first stage of ejaculation from occurring. Kedia and Markland (1975), however, found no evidence of retrograde ejaculation following extensive retroperitoneal lymphadenectomy.

Chemical sympathectomy resulting in retrograde ejaculation has been reported in patients receiving adrenergic blocking agents such as guanethidine, reserpine, thioridazine hydrochloride, bretylium and bethanedine (Rowan 1965). Shader (1964) found this condition occurred in 23% of males on guanethidine for hypertension. Several researchers have suggested that the ductus deferens, ampulla and seminal vesicles are under adrenergic control via the adrenergic receptors (Gennser et al. 1969; Andaloro and Dube 1975; Stewart and Bargani 1976; Shader 1964). Kedia and Markland (1975) considered that adrenergic blocking agents might inhibit the contractibility of these structures and therefore produce, rather than retrograde ejaculation, aspermia as a result of failure of the first stage of ejaculation. It is possible that both mechanisms are operative in producing aspermia (see Figure 1).

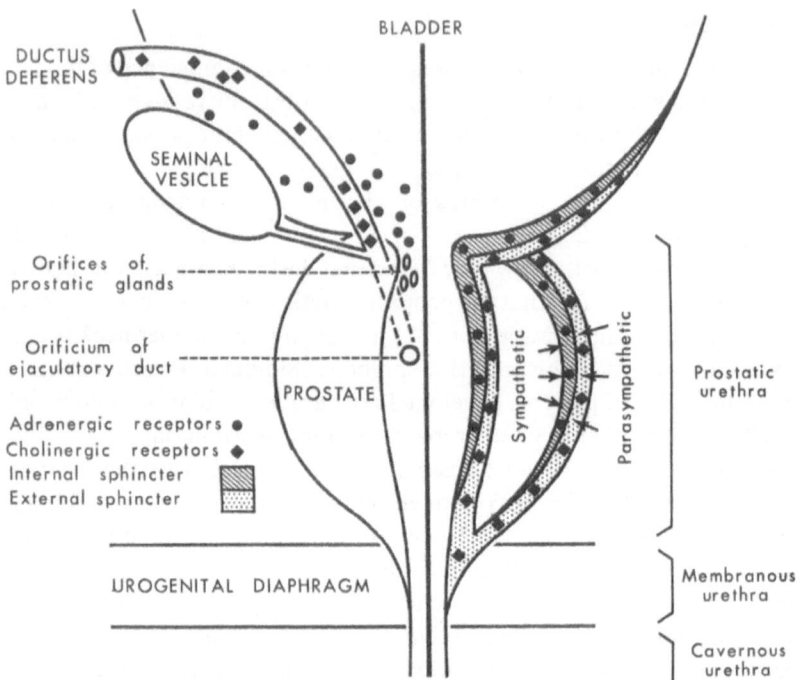

Figure 1. *Left:* relationship among the ductus deferens, seminal vesicle, and prostate and their outlets into the prostatic urethra. Note the dense adrenergic innervation of the bladder neck and cholinergic innervation of the ductus deferens and the seminal vesicle; *right:* topographic scheme of the internal and external sphincters.

4.2. Non-iatrogenic causes

The non-iatrogenic causes of retrograde ejaculation may be divided into congenital and acquired.

4.2.1. Congenital. A case of retrograde ejaculation in a patient with no apparent cause has been reported (Gennser et al. 1969). Investigation of the genitourinary system revealed aplasia of the right kidney, absence of the right testicle, a small prostate and an abnormal configuration of the proximal urethra. As the motor function of the bladder was normal and since the internal sphincter of the bladder is not distinct morphologically from the detrusor muscle, they concluded that the probable cause was a congenital defect of the sympathetic innervation of the internal sphincter.

4.2.2. Acquired. In reporting on 19 cases of retrograde ejaculation, Girgis and Etriby (1968) found five cases of long-standing urethral stricture. A tight urethral stricture may allow the passage of urine but not semen due to its greater viscosity. During erection the stricture becomes tighter and the semen is forced backwards, eventually leading to dilatation of the internal sphincter and retrograde ejaculation. Cystoscopy in these five cases revealed an atonic and dilated internal sphincter with visualization of the posterior urethra as far 'as the verumontanum.

In the same series a large bladder calculus was responsible in one patient. The presence of a large stone requires the patient to strain continuously during voiding and this may eventually lead to overstretching of the internal sphincter and ultimate loss of its ability to contract.

Retrograde ejaculation may also be produced by trauma to the spinal cord resulting in interruption of the sympathetic innervation of the internal sphincter (Kragt and Schellen 1978).

The association of retrograde ejaculation and diabetes mellitus was first noticed by Greene and Kelalis (1968). The most likely etiologic factor responsible in diabetes is dysfunction of the sympathetic innervation of the internal sphincter, since it has been shown that the sympathetic nervous system may be affected by diabetic neuropathy.

An unusual form of retrograde ejaculation was described by Keiserman et al. (1974). They reported three cases in which there was antegrade ejaculation of the initial sperm-free portion of the ejaculate and a retrograde ejaculation of the sperm-rich fraction which also contains fructose from the seminal vesicles.

5. DIAGNOSIS OF RETROGRADE EJACULATION

The importance of a sperm analysis early in the couple's fertility assessment is demonstrated by the fact that 40-50% of infertility problems rest with the male. Absence of ejaculate makes it mandatory to assess a postcoital urinary specimen for spermatozoa. The diagnosis of retrograde ejaculation is made by history and examination of the urine obtained after coitus or masturbation. In most patients the sensation of the ejaculation is retained but discharge of the semen does not occur. On urine analysis large numbers of immobile spermatozoa are present.

As previously mentioned three cases of retrograde ejaculation have been reported where partial antegrade ejaculation was present (Keiserman et al. 1974). These men had a low semen volume, azoospermia and absence of fructose from the seminal fluid. It is therefore important to assess a post-ejaculatory urine specimen in all such cases.

6. MANAGEMENT

It is wise to mention at this point that the successful treatment of retrograde ejaculation also depends on a thorough evaluation of female fertility. Thus cervical mucus assessment, hysterosalpingography, basal body temperature chart, and timed endometrial biopsy to demonstrate adequate luteal function, are important before definitive treatment of retrograde ejaculation is instituted.

Treatment of such cases may be of two kinds: (a) procedures to restore antegrade ejaculation, and (b) procedures to obtain viable and fertile sperm from the urinary bladder with subsequent artificial insemination.

6.1. Procedures to restore antegrade ejaculation

Restoration of antegrade ejaculation may be achieved by surgical or medical means. Successful surgical restoration has been reported in two patients. It is important to note that the cause of the condition in both patients was previous bladder neck surgery (Y-V-plasty of the bladder neck) and that surgery is not indicated in such conditions as diabetic neuropathy or urethral strictures.

The surgical technique to reconstruct the internal vesicle sphincter is performed transvesically. A 16F Foley catheter is passed per urethra. A long anterior cystotomy is performed to provide adequate exposure of the vesical neck. An inverted-U incision is made through the mucosa, beginning at the 8-o'clock position and continuing around the vesical neck to the 4-o'clock position. The mucosa is elevated approximately 1 cm into the prostatic urethra and excised. Using sharp dissection the underlying scar tissue is removed and the bladder neck muscle is exposed. The repair is made using H sutures of zero chromic catgut and joining the two links of the inverted U. The exposed muscle is approximately anterior to the Foley catheter, thus reconstructing the internal sphincter to a diameter of the 16F catheter. Closure is then achieved and the perivesical space is drained. The Foley catheter is removed 21 days later.

The successful use of α-adrenergic drugs in correcting retrograde ejaculation has been reported (Andaloro and Dube 1975; Budd 1975; Kedia and Markland 1975; Schirren and Hupe 1976). As previously mentioned the bladder neck is under sympathetic control and its receptor sites are of the α-type. It is logical, therefore, to attempt to correct the problem with medications that stimulate α-adrenergic receptor sites. Stockamp et al. (1974) reported the use of synephrine in a patient who had previously undergone a retroperitoneal lymphadenectomy because of malignant testicular teratoma with resultant retrograde ejaculation. Alpha-adrenergic drugs (synephrine) reversed the retrograde ejaculation resulting in normal sperm counts. This effect is attributable to an increase of bladder neck tone with consequent prevention of backflow of semen into the bladder. Phen-propranolamine (Ornade) produced an immediate increase in semen volume upon ejaculation and an increase in normal cell counts, motility and morphology (Stewart and Bargani 1976).

Brompheniramine, a drug with antihistaminic and anticholinergic properties has been reported to restore antegrade ejaculation in a juvenile diabetic (Anda-loro and Dube 1975). However, in spite of restoration of antegrade ejaculation, no pregnancy has been reported following pharmacologic treatment. The only successful method of treatment of infertility in such cases has been artificial insemination of the wife with the husband's semen (AIH) recovered from the bladder.

Whether retrograde ejaculation secondary to various neuropathic disorders or prostate surgery can be influenced pharmacologically in the same manner remains to be seen.

The absence of urine in the bladder at ejaculation has been repeatedly stressed (Kimura et al. 1975; Potts 1957), as urine, especially that of low osmolarity, has a rapid and profound effect on sperm motility (Crich and Jequier 1978). Erich and Jequier (1978) reported on two patients in which ejaculation was recommended on a full bladder, resulting in an antegrade sperm-rich semen only minimally contaminated with urine. However no pregnancies resulted. Two pregnancies have been reported using the post-ejaculate voiding technique, provided the urine is alkalined one day prior to the anticipated ovulation day of the wife (Schram 1976). The husband is advised to restrict fluids 6-8 hours prior to coitus. The couple are advised to have intercourse 'as usual' followed by post-ejaculation voiding directly into the vagina as soon as the husband is able to void.

6.2. AIH of recovered sperm from the urinary bladder after retrograde ejaculation

The standard treatment for retrograde ejaculation has been the use of artificial insemination of bladder contents after manually induced ejaculation (Amelar 1966). A pregnancy was reported with this technique, but the specimen was allowed to stay intact rather than centrifuged, to 'avoid injuring the sperm' (Walters and Kaufman 1959).

The technique used for collection of semen was basically the same as that described by Hotchkiss et al. (1955). The bladder was completely emptied by catheterization, using a No. 14 French catheter, and washed with 250 ml of 5% dextrose in lactated Ringer's solution. Manually induced ejaculation was immediately performed and the specimen was removed by another catheter (No. 14 French). The specimen was then centrifuged for three minutes and part of the sediment was inseminated. The remainder of the semen was preserved by freezing, using glycerol as a cryoprotective agent. Insemination of the freeze-preserved specimen was performed at the expected time of ovulation (Barwin 1974; Barwin and Beck 1976).

The technique of semen recovery from the bladder is time-consuming and uncomfortable to the patient, while the quality of the semen recovered is variable and the risk of iatrogenic bladder infection is increased (Fisher and Coats 1954). To avoid the above problems and to have sperm available for AIH at the time of ovulation the freeze-preserved ejaculate may be used for future AIH.

Due to the difficulty in precise timing of ovulation a number of inseminations may be required during the ovulatory phase (Barwin 1974). Having preserved semen available makes repeated AIH logistically feasible (Barwin and Beck 1976). Furthermore since acids are spermatocidal the urine into which the sperm is ejaculated should be alkaline (Crich and Jequier 1978; Fisher and Coats 1954). The use of adequate doses of bicarbonate to alkalinize the urine depends on many variables so the urine should be tested with nitrazine paper. Catheterization of the male immediately after intercourse or masturbation is a very traumatic procedure and easily flares up latent infection (Fisher and Coats 1954). It would therefore seem best to obtain the specimen by voiding.

A review of reported pregnancies achieved with AIH and retrograde ejaculate shows that the infertility was secondary to the male factor and that the fertility of all the wives was normal (Amelar 1966). Conceptions in all cases, in spite of the wives' normal fertility, occurred after multiple insemination which required repeated semen recovery from the bladder or postmasturbation or postcoital collection of semen (Table 1). Repeated inseminations were in most cases dictated by the unpredictable quality of the semen recovered and the unpredictability of ovulation. Repeated catheterization may result in bladder infection, so the advantage of post-voiding samples and sperm freezing is apparent. Sperm recovery following freezing and thawing of the recovered ejaculate was comparable to that observed with normal specimens (Kapetanakis et al. 1978; Barwin 1974).

7. CONCLUSIONS

Retrograde ejaculation, an infrequent cause of male infertility, may be the sequel of prostate or bladder neck surgery or the result of interruption in the sympathetic innervation to the bladder neck. The diagnosis is established by history and examination of the urine.

Temporary return of normal ejaculation has been achieved with adrenergic drugs, which increase bladder neck tone and prevent semen flow into the bladder in cases due to sympathetic nerve injury. In spite of restoration of antegrade ejaculation, no pregnancy has been reported following pharmacologic treatment.

In infertile couples artificial insemination homologous (AIH) using retrograde ejaculate recovered from the bladder has been successfully accomplished, but conception has occurred only in isolated cases. A literature review of the subject is presented.

Catheterization of the male immediately after intercourse is a very traumatic procedure and easily flares up latent infection. It would, therefore, seem best to

Table 1. Reported cases of conception after insemination (AIH) with retrograde ejaculate recovered from the bladder.

Etiology of retrograde ejaculation	Procedure/times repeated	Outcome	Authors
Transurethral surgery	AIH with bladder aspirate × 3 and with voided specimen × 4	Spontaneous abortion at 7 weeks	Fisher and Coats (1954)
Same patient as above 2 mo later	AIH with voided specimen × 12	Intrauterine pregnancy	Fisher and Coats (1954)
Transurethral prostatectomy	AIH with voided specimen × 3	Intrauterine pregnancy	Hotchkiss et al. (1955)
Same patient as above 2 mo later	AIH with voided specimen × 1	Intrauterine pregnancy	Hotchkiss et al. (1955)
Prostatic hypertrophy	AIH with voided specimen × 16	Intrauterine pregnancy	Hotchkiss et al. (1955)
Transurethral prostatectomy	AIH with voided specimen × 2	Intrauterine pregnancy	Walters and Kaufman (1959)
Diabetes mellitus	AIH with voided specimen × 14	Intrauterine pregnancy	Bourne et al. (1971)
Spinal cord injury	AIH with voided specimen × 15	Intrauterine pregnancy	Glezerman et al. (1976)
Transurethral surgery	AIH with voided specimen × (?)	Intrauterine pregnancy	Glezerman et al. (1976)
Transurethral surgery	AIH with voided specimen × 2	Midtrimester abortion	Kapetanakis (1978)
Transurethral surgery	AIH × 12*	Intrauterine pregnancy	
Transurethral surgery	AIH × 4	Intrauterine pregnancy	
Spinal cord injury	AIH × 8	Intrauterine pregnancy	
Spinal cord injury	AIH × 12*	Intrauterine pregnancy	Present series
Retroperitoneal surgery	AIH × 7	Normal delivery	
Retroperitoneal surgery	AIH × 3*	Intrauterine pregnancy	
Diabetic neuropathy	AIH × 5	Aborted	

* Freeze-preserved.

collect the specimen by voiding.

In order to have sperm available at ovulation and due to the variable quality of sperm recovery freeze-preserved ejaculate is recommended.

REFERENCES

Amelar RD: General considerations. In: *Infertility in men: diagnosis and treatment*, Philadelphia, Davis, 1966, p 25.
Andaloro VA, Dube A: Treatment of retrograde ejaculation with brompheniramine. *Urology* 5:520, 1975.
Barwin BN: Intrauterine insemination of husband's semen. *J Reprod Fertil* 36:101, 1974.
Barwin BN, Beck WW: Artificial insemination and semen preservation. In: *Human semen and fertility regulation in men*, Hafez ESE (ed), St. Louis, Mosby 1976, p 429.
Bol JJ: Successful artificial insemination with spermatozoa recovered from the urine in a case of retrograde ejaculation. *Eur J Obst Gyn Repr Biol* 3:89-92, 1973.
Bourne RB, Kretzschmar WA, Esser JH: Successful artificial insemination in a diabetic with retrograde ejaculation. *Fertil Steril* 22:275, 1971.
Budd HA: Brompheniramine in the treatment of retrograde ejaculation. *Urology* 6:131, 1975.
Crich JP, Jequier AM: Infertility in men with retrograde ejaculation: the action of urine on sperm motility, and a simple method for achieving antegrade ejaculation. *Fertil Steril* 30:572, 1978.
Fisher I, Coats E: Sterility due to retrograde ejaculation of semen. *Obstet Gynecol* 4:352, 1954.
Gennser G, Owman C. Owman T, Wehlin L: Significance of adrenergic innervation of the bladder outlet during ejaculation. *Lancet* 1:184, 1969.
Girgis SM, Etriby A, El-Hefnawy H, Kahil SL: Aspermia: a survey of 49 cases. *Fertil Steril* 19:580, 1968.
Glezerman M, Lunenfeld B, Potashnik G, Oelsner G, Beer R: Retrograde ejaculation: pathophysiologic aspects and report of two successfully treated cases. *Fertil Steril* 27:796, 1976.
Goligher JC: Sexual function after excision of the rectum. *Proc Roy Soc Med* 44:824, 1951.
Greene LF, Kelalis PP: Retrograde ejaculation of semen due to diabetic neuropathy. *J Urol* 98:693, 1968.
Hollister L: Drugs and sexual behaviour in man. *Life Sci* 17:661-668, 1976.
Hotchkiss RS, Pinto AB, Kleegman S: Artificial insemination with semen recovered from the bladder. *Fertil Steril* 6:37, 1955.
Innes-Williams D, Watson PC, Goligher JC, Riches EW, Gabriel WD, Pyrah LN: Discussion of urological complications of excision of the rectum. *Proc Roy Soc Med* 44:819, 1950-1951.
Kapetanakis E, Rao R, Dmowski WP, Scommegna A: Conception following insemination with a freeze-preserved retrograde ejaculate. *Fertil Steril* 29:360, 1978.
Kedia K, Markland C: The effect of pharmacological agents on ejaculation. *J Urol* 114:569, 1975.
Keiserman WM, Dubin L, Amelar RD: A new type of retrograde ejaculation: report of three cases. *Fertil Steril* 25:1071, 1974.
Kimura Y, Miyata K, Adachi K, Kisaki N: Peripheral nerves controlling the closure of internal urethral orifice during ejaculation. *Urol Int* 30:218-227, 1975.
Kragt F, Schellen A: Clinical report about some cases with retrograde ejaculation. *Andrologia* 10:381, 1978.
Leiter E, Brendler H: Loss of ejaculation following bilateral retroperitoneal lymphadenectomy. *J Urol* 98:375, 1967.
Ochsner MG, Burns E, Henry HH: Incidence of retrograde ejaculation following bladder neck revision as a child. *J Urol* 104:596, 1970.
Potts IF: The mechanism of ejaculation. *Med J Aust* 1:495, 1957.
Retieff PJM: Physiology of micturition and ejaculation. *S African Med J* 24:509, 1950.
Rieser C: The etiology of retrograde ejaculation and method for insemination. *Fertil Steril* 12:488-492, 1961.
Rowan RL, Howley TF: Ejaculatory sterility. *Fertil Steril* 16:768, 1965.
Schellen TMCM: A case of retrograde ejaculation caused by a colon operation. *Fertil Steril* 11-187, 1960.
Schirren C, Hupe H: Immer daran denken: retrograde Ejakulation. *Urologe* B16:108-110, 1976.
Schram JD: Retrograde ejaculation: a new approach to therapy. *Fertil Steril* 27:1216, 1976.
Shader RI: Sexual dysfunction associated with thioridazine hydrochloride. *JAMA* 188:1007, 1964.

Stewart BH, Bargani JA: Correction of retrograde ejaculation by sympathomimetic medication: preliminary report. *Fertil Steril* 27:1215, 1976.

Stockamp K, Schreiter F, Altwein JE: Alpha-adrenergic drugs in retrograde ejaculation. *Fertil Steril* 25:817, 1974.

Walters D, Kaufman MS: Sterility due to retrograde ejaculation of semen. *Am J Obstet Gynecol* 78:274, 1959.

13. AIH WITH FREEZE-PRESERVED RETROGRADE EJACULATE

W.P. Dmowski, E. Kapetanakis, R. Rao and A. Scommegna

Male factors, either absolute or relative may be the cause of infertility in about 40% of childless couples (Speroff et al. 1975). Retrograde ejaculation into the urinary bladder, a result of inadequate closure of the internal sphincter of the urethra, is an infrequent cause of male infertility but during recent years its incidence appears to be on the increase (Schram 1976).

1. PHYSIOLOGY OF NORMAL EJACULATION

Normal ejaculation is a complex reflex action mediated through the central nervous system and occurring in four phases: erection, emission, formation of pressure chamber, and expulsion of semen (Marberger 1974). Emission begins with peristaltic contractions of the smooth muscles surrounding the ducts of the testis, the epididymis and the vas deferens and causing expulsion of the sperm into the prostatic urethra. Simultaneously, rhythmic contractions of the seminal vesicles and prostate expel seminal and prostatic fluid along with the sperm as the semen.

Emission of the semen into the posterior urethra is the trigger impulse for the next phase of the ejaculation. The pressure chamber forms in the posterior urethra and in response to sympathetic nervous system stimulation, smooth muscles around the bladder neck contract, preventing the semen from entering the bladder. Simultaneously, the external sphincter is relaxed by parasympathetic activity allowing antegrade propulsion of the semen, which is facilitated by rhythmic contractions of the urethral constrictor, bulbocavernosus, ischiocavernosus and other associated perineal muscles. The stimulus initiating contractions of the striated muscles is transmitted by somatic nerves.

2. PATHOPHYSIOLOGY OF RETROGRADE EJACULATION

Incomplete closure of the vesical neck favors retrograde ejaculation through the path of least resistance. Any condition which interferes with the anatomical properties of the bladder neck or interrupts sympathetic innervation of the lower urinary tract may result in abnormal function of the sphincter and may cause retrograde ejaculation. Some of the common causes of retrograde ejaculation are listed in Table 1.

In males of reproductive age the most common cause of retrograde ejaculation is transurethral surgical resection of the bladder neck (Ochsner et al. 1970) or prostate (Rieser 1961), which interrupts the continuity of the internal sphincter. However, retrograde ejaculation may also be the result of interruption of the sympathectomy (Rose 1953), or abdominal-perineal resection (Goligher 1951). Peripheral diabetic neuropathy may be another cause of retrograde ejaculation Peripheral diabetic neuropathy may be another cause of retrograde ejaculation but it is generally seen at a later age (Ellenberg and Weber 1966; Greene and Kelaris 1967). Reversible retrograde ejaculation has been observed in patients on antihypertensive drugs such as guanethidine (Ismelin), with sympathetic nerve-blocking properties (Shirger and Gifford 1962). In such cases antegrade ejaculation resumes within two weeks of discontinuation of the medication.

Table 1. Etiology of retrograde ejaculation.

A. *Mechanical disruption of the internal sphincter of the bladder neck and posterior urethra*
  1. Hypertrophy, inflammation or tumor of the prostate
  2. Prostatic and bladder neck surgery
  3. Sclerosis of the bladder neck
  4. Congenital malfunction and strictures of the urethra

B. *Interruption of sympathetic innervation*
  1. Surgical or chemical sympathectomy
  2. Trauma to the spinal cord
  3. Radical retroperitoneal lymphadenectomy
  4. Deep pelvic dissection
  5. Diabetic neuropathy
  6. Congenital

3. DIAGNOSIS AND TREATMENT OF RETROGRADE EJACULATION

The diagnosis of retrograde ejaculation is made by history and examination of the urine obtained after coitus or masturbation. In most patients the sensation of the ejaculation is retained but discharge of the semen does not occur. On urinalysis large numbers of immobile sperms are present.

Treatment of retrograde ejaculation is indicated only in individuals interested in fertility. Temporary return of normal ejaculation has been achieved with adrenergic drugs, which increase bladder neck tone and prevent semen flow into the bladder in cases due to sympathetic nerve injury (Stockamp et al. 1974; Stewart and Bergant 1974). Brompheniramine, a drug with antihistaminic and

Table 2. Reported cases of conception after insemination (AIH) with retrograde ejaculate recovered from the bladder.

No.	Etiology of retrograde ejaculation	Wife's Fertility	Procedure/ times repeated	Outcome	Author	Comments
1.	Transurethral surgery	Normal	AIH with bladder aspirate × 3 and with voided specimen × 4	Spontaneous abortion 7 weeks	Fisher and Coats (1954)	Severe bladder infection after catheterization
2.	The same patient as above two months later	Normal	AIH with voided specimen × 12	Intrauterine pregnancy	Fisher and Coats (1954)	Catheterization was omitted to avoid UTI
3.	Transurethral prostatectomy	Normal	AIH with voided specimen × 3	Intrauterine pregnancy	Hotchkiss et al. (1954	Variability in semen quality
4.	The same patient as above two months later	Normal	AIH with voided specimen × 1	Intrauterine pregnancy	Hotchkiss et al. (1954)	
5.	Prostatic hypertrophy	Normal	AIH with voided specimen × 16	Intrauterine pregnancy	Hotchkiss et al. (1954)	Variability in semen quality
6.	Transurethral prostatectomy	Normal	AIH with voided specimen × 2	Intrauterine pregnancy	Walters and Kaufman (1959)	
7.	Diabetes mellitus	Normal	AIH with voided specimen × 14	Intrauterine pregnancy	Bourne et al. 1971	Variability in semen quality
8.	Spinal cord injury	Normal	AIH with voided specimen × 15	Intrauterine pregnancy	Glezerman et al. (1976)	Prophylactic antibiotics for UTI
9.	Transurethral surgery	Normal	AIH with voided specimen × (?)	Intrauterine pregnancy	Glezerman et al. (1976)	Variability in semen quality
10.	Transurethral surgery	Anovulation	AIH with voided specimen × 2; Clomid + HCG + AIH with freeze-preserved voided specimen × 3	Mid-trimester abortion	Kapetanakis et al. (1978)	Husband with history of re-current UTI

anticholinergic properties has been reported to restore antegrade ejaculation in a juvenile diabetic (Andaloro and Dube 1954). However, in spite of restoration of antegrade ejaculation, no pregnancy has been reported following pharmacological treatment. The only successful method of treatment of infertility in such cases has been insemination of the wife with husband's semen recovered from the bladder (AIH). A review of the published cases of AIH pregnancies achieved with retrograde ejaculate (Table 2) shows that infertility was secondary to the male factor and that fertility of all spouses was normal (Fisher and Coats 1954; Hotchkiss et al. 1955; Walters and Kaufman 1959; Glezerman et al. 1976; Bourne et al. 1971).

Conceptions in all cases, in spite of the wife's normal fertility, occurred after multiple inseminations which required repeated semen recovery from the bladder. The necessity for repeated inseminations was in most cases dictated by the unpredictable quality of semen recovered.

Repeated bladder catheterizations, a part of the technique of semen recovery, were contributory to the development of urinary tract infection in at least three cases. In at least one case (case 1 in Table 2) this complication was severe enough to interfere with the semen recovery procedure.

If retrograde ejaculation in the husband is combined with anovulation or erratic ovulation in the wife, more frequent inseminations may be necessary, thus further complicating the problem. In order to avoid repeated bladder catheterizations and yet still have semen available for insemination when needed, we elected to freeze-preserve good-quality semen recovered from the bladder for subsequent insemination of the oligo-ovulatory wife.

4. CONCEPTION FOLLOWING AIH WITH A FREEZE-PRESERVED RETROGRADE EJACULATE

The infertile couple had both male and female contributory factors to their infertility. The 42-year-old husband developed retrograde ejaculation subsequent to surgery for bladder neck obstruction, eight years prior to the initial visit. He had frequent bouts of urinary tract infection, for which he was treated with antibiotics. The 37-year old-wife had oligomenorrhea since menarche. Unpredictable and infrequent ovulations were diagnosed during the infertility assessment. Recovery of the ejaculate from the bladder was performed about the expected time of ovulation using a modification of the Hotchkiss technique (Bourne et al. 1971), the principles of which are outlined in Table 3.

The volume of recovered semen was 3.5 cc. The sperm count was 100×10^6 per cc with 70% motility and 70% normal forms. Part of the specimen was used for insemination of the wife, and part was preserved by freezing. The technique used for freeze preservation of the semen is shown in Table 4. During subsequent

Table 3. Retrograde ejaculation: technique of semen recovery for AIH.

1. Alkalinization of the urine, $NaHCO_3$, 3.6 gm P.O. evening before and morning of semen recovery

2. Irrigation of the bladder: irrigate bladder with 5% D in Ringer's lactate; leave 2 cc of the solution in the bladder

3. Recovery of the semen: after ejaculation, recover bladder contents by voiding or catheterization if needed (specimen may have to be centrifuged at 3,400 rpm × 3 min if needed)

4. Insemination (AIH) with recovered specimen

Table 4. Technique for freeze-preservation of semen

1. Collect the specimen in a jar and measure total volume
2. Check sperm count and motility
3. Add glycerol dropwise to a concentration of 7.5%
4. Allow equilibration of specimen and glycerol for 20 minutes
5. Fill plastic straws with specimen (approximately 0.5 cc/straw) and seal open ends.
6. Place straws for 20 minutes in liquid nitrogen vapor tank ($-75°C$)
7. Transfer straws into liquid nitrogen tank for storage ($-196°C$)

cycles the wife's ovulation was induced with clomiphene and HCG. Inseminations with freeze-preserved specimen were performed at the time of expected ovulation (Figure 1). Conception occurred in the second cycle of ovulation induction or fourth cycle of AIH. Only two ejaculate recovery procedures were performed. Sperm recovery following freezing and thawing of the recovered ejaculate was comparable to that observed with normal specimens (Beck 1974).

There was immediate loss of about 45% motility after freezing and thawing. Subsequently however, sperm recovery remained stable for about 40 weeks of storage, varying between 30-45% of original motility (Figure 2).

In summary we can conclude that semen from retrograde ejaculation recovered from the bladder may be freeze-preserved and stored for subsequent AIH.

The advantage of this technique over direct insemination with retrograde ejaculate is clear when the wife's ovulation is unpredictable. However, even if the wife has normal fertility, this technique can facilitate storage of at least a part of the specimen for future use, thus minimizing the risk of repeated catheterizations.

THREE CYCLES

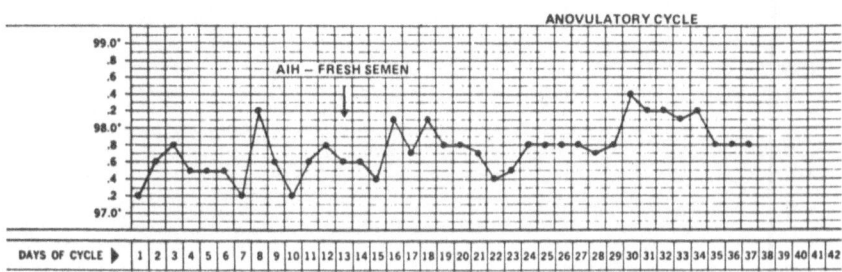

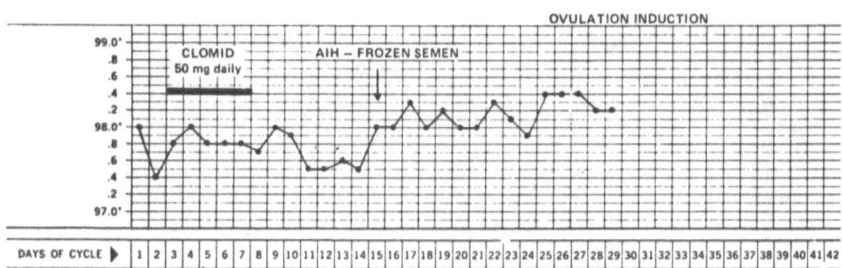

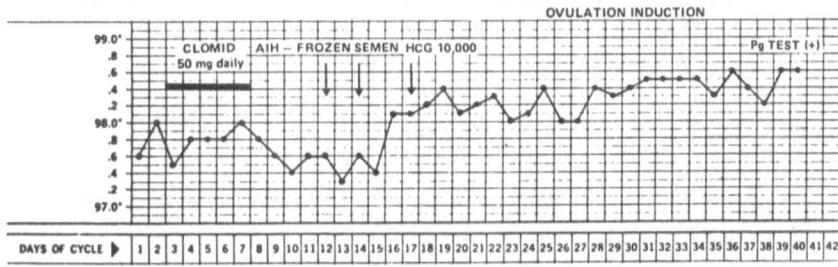

Figure 1. Three cycles of AIH with retrograde ejaculate in an anovulatory wife, Fresh specimen was used during the first, anovulatory cycle and freeze-preserved semen recovered from the bladder in the other two cycles. Ovulation was induced with Clomid in the second and Clomid and HCG in the third cycle. Conception occurred in the third cycle of treatment.

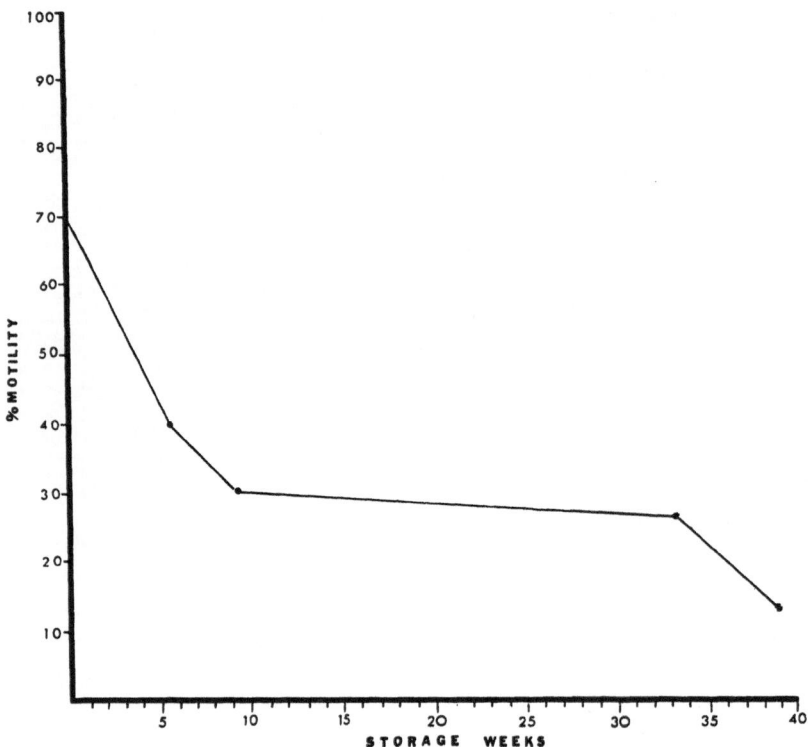

Figure 2. Original and post-thaw motility of semen recovered from the bladder, freeze-preserved and stored in liquid nitrogen.

REFERENCES

Andaloro V, Dube A: Treatment of retrograde ejaculation with brompheniramine. *Urology* 5:520, 1975.

Beck WW: Artificial insemination and semen preservation. *Clin Obstet Gynecol* 17:115, 1974.

Bourne RB, Kretzschmar WA, Esser JH: Successful artificial insemination in a diabetic with retrograde ejaculation. *Fertil Steril* 22:275, 1971.

Ellenberg M. Weber H: Retrograde ejaculation in diabetic neuropathy. *Ann Int. Med* 65: 1237, 1966.

Fisher I, Coats E: Sterility due to retrograde ejaculation of semen. *Obstet Gynecol* 4:352, 1954.

Glezerman M, Lunenfeld B, Potashnik G, Oelsrier G, Beer R: Retrograde ejaculation: pathophysiologic aspects and report of two successfully treated cases. *Fertil Steril* 27: 796, 1976.

Goligher JC: Sexual function after excision of the rectum. *Proc Roy Soc Med* 44:824, 1951.

Greene LF, Kelalis PP: Retrograde ejaculation of semen due to diabetic neuropathy. *J Urol* 98:693, 1967.

Hotchkiss RS, Pinto AB, Kleegman S: Artificial insemination with semen recovered from the bladder. *Fertil Steril* 6:37, 1955.

Kapetanakis E, Rao R, Dmowski WP, Scommegna A: Conception following insemination with a freeze-preserved retrograde ejaculate. *Fertil Steril* 29:360, 1978.

Marberger H: The mechanisms of ejaculation. *Basic Life Sci* 4 (B):99, 1974.

Ochsner MG, Burns E, Henry HH: Incidence of retrograde ejaculation following bladder neck revision as a child. *J Urol* 104:596, 1970.

Rieser C: The etiology of retrograde ejaculation and a method of insemination. *Fertil Steril* 12:488, 1961.

Rose S: An investigation into sterility after lumbar ganglionectomy. *Brit Med J* 247, 1953.

Schram JD: Retrograde ejaculation: a new approach to therapy. *Fertil Steril* 27:1216, 1976.

Shirger A, Gifford RW: Guanethidine, a new antihypertensive agent: experience in the treatment of 36 patients with severe hypertension. *Proc Mayo Clin* 37:100, 1962.

Speroff L, Glass HR, Kase GN: *Clinical gynecologic endocrinology and infertility*, Williams and Wilkins, 1975,

Stewart BH, Bergant JA: Correction of retrograde ejaculation by sympathomimetic medication: preliminary report. *Fertil Steril* 25:1073, 1974.

Stockamp K, Schreiter F, Altwein JE: α-adrenergic drugs in retrograde ejaculation. *Fertil Steril* 25:817, 1974.

Walters D, Kaufman MS: Sterility due to retrograde ejaculation of semen. *Am J Obstet Gynecol* 78:274, 1959.

14. CRYOBANKING OF SEMEN IN AIH

J.K. SHERMAN

Artificial or therapeutic insemination of the wife with husband or homologous semen, referred to as AIH, is an established worldwide practice in reproductive medicine. The extent of AIH, although unknown in terms of numbers, is much less than insemination involving donor or heterologous semen (AID). It is used, however, to some degree in most subfertility or infertility clinics as well as by physicians specializing in problems of reproduction.

Cryopreservation is that branch of cryobiology which is concerned with the indefinite prolongation of the potential life span of cells by reversible suspension of biochemical activity through ice formation at extremely low, sub-freezing temperatures. It is the antithesis of cryosurgery which is directed toward the killing of cells by their exposure to the formation and dissolution of ice. Cryobanks are the vehicles used to realize the clinical and research applications of cryopreserved cells and tissues.

1. HISTORY OF SEMEN CRYOBANKING

Highlights in the historical development of low-temperature research and cryobanking of human semen are detailed and referenced elsewhere (Sherman 1973, 1977). The concept of cryobanks for human semen was first proposed in 1866. It was the accidental discovery and subsequent use of the polyhydric alcohol, glycerol, as a cryoprotective agent, however, which initiated the establishment of banks for frozen mammalian spermatozoa. Emphasis was placed at first on the economically important semen of farm animals, especially the bull. It was not until 1953-1954 that a successful, practical technique for cryopreservation of human spermatozoa was introduced along with the demonstration that the spermatozoa, after being frozen and stored in dry ice ($-78°$ C) were capable of fertilization and the subsequent induced development of normal progeny. In the following decade only about 25 births were reported in the United States and Japan, all but one from the use of cryopreserved donor semen. This relative inactivity in cryobanking was due perhaps in part to methods, but certainly to physicians who were not ready for evaluative application in an atmosphere of relative uncertainty, even about the practice of insemination itself. The introduction in 1963-1964 of a method for freezing human semen in the vapor of liquid nitrogen and its storage at $-196°$ C was accompanied by realization of normal births with its use. Later, positive research findings were presented which supported the safety and efficacy of frozen storage of human spermatozoa. Greater appreciation of the applications of cryobanking developed with the wider use of AID and AIH. Warnings from panels of the American Public Health Association and Planned Parenthood-World Population, which were based on incompletely researched evaluation, however, did much to inhibit development. The establishment of much-publicized commercial cryobanks in about 1972 was based primarily on the reasonable expectation that millions of men would elect to store their semen as 'fertility insurance' prior to undergoing vasectomy in population control. This has since proved to be an unrealized expectation, the economically important absence of which has slowed considerably the growth of commercial banking. There are about a dozen commercial and university-based banks in the United States, about thirteen national banks in France (David 1975), and probably fewer than ten other cryobanks throughout the rest of the world, including Austria, Israel and Brazil. Based on incomplete surveys and personal contacts, with full appreciation of limitations in coverage, an estimate of over 5,000 births from the clinical use of frozen stored human semen is considered conservative. Normal births have resulted from semen stored for over ten years, and there is no evidence of mutagenic effects of cryobanking. To the contrary, the percentage of abnormal progeny is considerably below that of the normal population. Even the abortion rate appears slightly below the normal level. Emphasis today is still on cryobanking for AID, but the recent awakening interest in certain applications of AIH with unique related benefits of cryobanking has stimulated more activity in AIH with cryobanked human semen in both research evaluation and the clinical practice of infertility. It has also emphasized the limitations of semen quality in realizing the potential afforded by these applications in infertility therapy, along with the coincident need for improving upon both the quality of semen used for AIH and the attendant methods for its frozen storage.

Successful cryobanking extends and enriches the attributes of artificial (therapeutic) insemination of fresh semen in infertility therapy and population control to include:

A. Timed multiple insemination of husband semen (AIH) or donor semen (AID) to coincide better with irregular female cycles or special conditions of the female tract, with the same or naturally optimal numbers of spermatozoa;

B. Storage, pooling and concentration of oligospermic samples of the husband to increase numbers of motile cells inseminated in AIH;

C. Storage of spermatozoa, whose quality is first improved by *in vitro* treatments, for more potentially fertile use later in AIH;

D. Retention of fertilizing capacity of husband or donor even in his temporary or permanent absence;

E. Therapeutic substitution of donor semen for the infertile husband in various timed protocols, on demand;

F. Production of a family of progeny from the same donor throughout a period of years, on demand, without the donor;

G. Wide selection of donor semen and ready availability favor practice of the concept of germinal choice by a couple to improve upon the genetic attributes of the population;

H. Restriction of the number of births by encouraging vasectomy after banking of semen for possible future AIH in retention of fertilizing capacity.

2. PURPOSE OF PRESENTATION

Appreciation of the actual and potential role of cryobanking of human semen in AIH depends upon an assessment of the historical and current applications of AIH with fresh semen. It also requires information as to the possibilities for the enhancement and extension of AIH by recent research advances in andrology which can be implemented by cryopreservation of spermatozoa. The purpose of this overview is to update the status of both AIH and cryobanking relative to current and prospective relationships between the two in reproductive biology. It is not possible to present this subject as a scientific discourse. There are essentially no hard data on the interrelated aspects of cryopreservation and reproductive function with which one can discuss figures, percentages, mechanisms and comparisons with authority and agreement among investigators. Indeed, based upon the extent of clinical practice, there is a paucity of definitive results in therapeutic insemination itself, for both fresh and frozen semen from either husband or donor. An attempt will be made to illustrate this situation with the differences and difficulties encountered in the evaluation of AIH with fresh semen. This dilemma in the relationship between AIH and cryobanking will remain until a concerted effort is made by physicians, especially, to document more completely those cases which involve insemination with frozen-stored semen, especially in carefully designed investigations. It is hoped, also, that efforts will be made by cryobiologists like myself to devote more time and to gain enough information to improve further upon the cryobanking methods in terms of functional survival of human spermatozoa in appropriate and beneficial clinical applications. In spite of our limitations, the subject is important enough to present here. Perhaps discussion of this brief presentation will stimulate greater use of cryobanking in AIH designed for more scientific evaluation and, therefore, a more rapid realization of its potential in favoring and improving the successful expression of man's fertility.

3. HISTORY OF AIH

The best source for details and references on the early history of AIH as well as AID is Schellen (1957). Insemination in the human in medical applications was initiated about two hundred years ago with husband, not donor, semen. Presumably, some time between 1776 and 1799, an English clinician, John Hunter, either performed himself or, more likely, directed a husband with hypospadias to perform a reproductively successful AIH with semen injected intravaginally from a warm syringe. This 'first' apparently went unnoticed by the medical world until the method was revived in France where publications in 1865 and 1868 revealed the successful and scientifically improved practice of AIH since 1838 by Girault. J. Marion Sims in 1866 reported the first series of cases and the first success of AIH in the United States, where he contributed a more thoughtful approach to both indication and technique. France continued to be most active, followed in time by Germany, while England was engaged quietly in AIH until its noteworthy emergence through a publication by Barton and associates in 1945. AID apparently was first used successfully, as late as 1884, by Pancost in Philadelphia, as reported in 1909.

The more recent history of AIH and AID reflects increased knowledge of reproductive physiology in the male and the female, as well as the widespread use of insemination as an accepted medical practice in aspects of infertility therapy. Until about the mid 1960's, however, most clinical experts and practitioners in the field of infertility concentrated on general medication for the oligospermic husbands rather than AIH or AID. Vitamins, testosterone, thyroid and other hormones were acceptable therapeutic agents. Results obviously were poor, and prognosis with these medications proved disappointing (Finegold 1976; Moghissi et al. 1977). Insemination has since become a more popular and clinically reliable substitute for medication and, when indicated and within its limitations, AIH has met the challenge of its applications. The degree of its success has varied with the particular application as well as with other factors including the complexity of evaluation in the comparison of clinical findings in its use.

4. APPLICATIONS OF AIH

AIH is applicable or indicated for clinical use under the following conditions:

1. When normal coitus is not possible or is not effective in terms of reproduction because of male or female inadequacies or abnormalities in physical, physiological or emotional factors in their system. These factors include:
   A. Defects which prevent the penetration of the ejaculate into the vagina, such as impotence, retrograde ejaculation, hypospadias, epispadias, vaginismus,

stenosis or atresia of the vagina, dyspareunia and marked obesity.
   B. Defects which prevent the penetration of spermatozoa into cervical mucus, as caused by largely unknown factors, immunological factors of semen and/or mucus, poor quality of motile spermatozoa, or all of these.
   C. Defects which prevent the penetration of spermatozoa into the cervix and uterus, as well as tumors, stenosis of cervix, prolapse of uterus.
2. When there is an infertile marriage of unknown cause or causes but with normal coitus.
3. When there are certain deficiencies or defects in production of semen, especially spermatozoa, such as oligospermia, asthenospermia, small volume, high viscosity, or a high percentage of structural abnormalities.
4. When there is clinical need to regulate ovulation by hormone therapy and to deliver semen at precise times to favor fertilization in treatment of subfertility.

5. EVALUATION OF AIH

The consensus is that AIH is indicated and is extremely effective in cases of infertility due either to inability to effect coitus or to failure to deliver a large enough volume, with otherwise normal or fertile semen. The literature reveals marked disagreement, however, when AIH is used for other reproductive deficiencies, especially those in number and/or motility of normal-appearing spermatozoa. There is a wide spectrum of reported rates of success in such applications, ranging from 0% to over 50%, which is reflected best by conclusions reached by experts in the field who either discourage or foster the practice.

In recent years there has been a tendency by some to regard AIH as valueless and even improper as a medical procedure when husband's semen is of questionable or poor quality, as evidenced by:

A. From a purely physiologic point of view, AIH has no advantage over coitus in treating sterility of undetermined origin and is of little value in sterility due to subnormal semen (Guttmacher 1960).

B. When semen quality is poor, there is no evidence that AIH improves chances of conception. There is as much chance of success in normal intercourse (Russel 1960), probably more as semen handling in AIH may reduce its fertilizing capacity (Guttmacher 1960).

C. Success rate with AIH has been 85% in cases of marital difficulty, but in cases of oligospermia or cervical impermeability results were poor. Various techniques to improve the rate of success with poor-quality semen, including the concentration of spermatozoa by centrifugation, were tried but with unsatisfactory results. AIH is of no value in cervical impermeability since the problem usually is basic infertility of the woman due to endocrine dysfunction (Kleegman and Kaufman 1966).

D. Results with oligospermia have been generally poor since a low sperm count is frequently associated with other morphological and biochemical abnormalities of the ejaculate (Moghissi et al. 1977).

E. Using four insemination methods and semen with various concentrations of spermatozoa, the conclusion is that AIH is useless in cases of oligospermia (Mastroianni et al. 1957).

F. AIH is useless if semen is inadequate in number and mobility and the outcome in attempts at circumventing oligospermia is poor, confirming reports of others (Warner 1974; Dixon et al. 1976; Speichinger and Mattox 1976; Harrison 1978).

In contrast to the dismal picture presented above, AIH is considered by some as a valuable clinical method in infertility therapy including conditions of oligospermia, asthenospermia, sperm antibodies, cervical hostility and retrograde ejaculation. The workers have concluded that:

A. Homologous insemination can be an important therapeutic tool in the treatment of infertility after careful selection of patients (Ulstein 1973).

B. AIH has a limited but important place in the management of childlessness (Russell 1960).

C. AIH is of value when cervical mucus is thick and refractory to hormone treatment or when the postcoital test repeatedly shows no spermatozoa or immotile spermatozoa (White and Glass 1976).

D. AIH is a useful mode of therapy in oligospermia and subfertility (Steiman and Taymor 1977).

E. The method of AIH is valuable even with oligospermia and reduced percentage motility (Usherwood et al. 1976).

F. AIH is successful in cases of poor semen quality, including oligospermia, with pregnancy rates of 50% (Janczewski 1975).

G. The method (AIH) has gained a stable place in the therapy of sterility, including the treatment of oligospermia and asthenospermia (Weller 1976).

H. When semen quality is borderline, with less than optimal sperm concentration or sperm motility, insemination with husband's spermatozoa may increase chances of pregnancy (Amelar et al. 1977).

I. A favorite treatment for oligospermia is the use of centrifugation to concentrate spermatozoa for AIH, with much better success than anticipated. AIH has become the vogue in treatment of infertility and enthusiasm for it is most deserving (Finegold 1976).

6. COMPLEXITY OF AIH EVALUATION

The evaluation of the effectiveness of AIH in the treatment of infertility or subfertility is controversial because it is extremely complicated and limited. This is true not only within the experience or practice of one physician or clinic, but also and especially in comparing results reported by individuals or groups in the literature. Reasons for this dilemma include:

A. The multiple factors related to the female's reproductive system, the quality of semen, as well as interactions between the two, are unique for each couple.

B. The number of variables in the possible factors affecting male and female fertility is so great, compared with the relatively low number of patients treated, that a true statistical analysis is essentially impossible.

C. There are inherent biological variations in patients and, especially, in characteristics of semen and its production and function, which often are undetected.

D. Many couples have multifaceted problems precluding the definition of a pure sample.

E. The experimental designs of evaluative studies, which most often are retrospective in data analysis relative to known factors compared, are frequently inadequately constructed.

F. Drugs are used to induce and control the timing of ovulation or to affect the production and motility of spermatozoa with some patients or series and not with others.

G. Both the length of the (number of trials), the number of early dropouts, and the recording of both as results often vary.

H. The medical assessment of the female and the male in the detection of factors of fertility may vary as to its depth, number, types and validity of measurements or observations.

I. The characteristics of the insemination technique may vary as to the technique itself (intrauterine, intravaginal, intracervical, cervical cap, etc.); the number and size of insemination units; as well as timing relative to ovulation.

J. The use of adjectives such as oligospermic, asthenospermic, good, poor, average, and the like, are applied especially to semen or spermatozoa, usually without accompanying definition.

K. The choice of procedures for measurements of the characteristics of the semen used and its treatment prior to insemination may be different.

L. The patients will vary in their previous medical history, especially with regard to therapy.

M. The skill, resourcefulness and perseverance of physicians are variables which remain undefined in publication.

N. Extramarital activity may further complicate efficacy of analysis of the results of particular regimes of therapy.

7. EXPERIENCE IN AIH

An unknown, modest number of physicians no doubt are using AIH with frozen as well as fresh semen, but most of them are not reporting their results at meetings or in the literature. They cannot be expected to present or to publish such data, however, if they are not in the habit of doing research or writing papers on other therapeutic procedures. Obviously, these physicians and others may not be reached by questionnaires because their activity in this infertility application is unknown. In addition, many of those individuals who receive questionnaires neglect to respond, respond with incomplete data, or fail to complete a follow-up inquiry. This is frustrating, at best, to those of us who attempt to gather this information because it is essential both for intelligent evaluation of progress to date and for the exchange of results requisite for research and clinical direction. Data in this field will remain sketchy and approximate unless specialty societies in reproductive biology, or those like the newly-founded American Association of Tissue Banks (AATB), can learn the identity of clinicians active in AIH and obtain their cooperation in providing data in the field, through a central vehicle like the Reproductive Council of the AATB, for a more authoritative dissemination to all.

A literature search by the author, however, reveals over 2,800 cases of AIH with fresh semen with a demonstrated pregnancy rate of about 20%. Approximately 75% of these cases were identified as male factor infertility directly associated with deficiencies in the quality of spermatozoa in the ejaculate. Data on pregnancies, not births, constituted the end point of fertility in the majority of cases. No subsequent reports have been seen on the results of pregnancies, however. There was insufficient data, therefore, to permit statistical treatment of results of AIH as to number and normalcy of progeny produced, percentage of spontaneous abortions, or any correlation of pregnancy rate with particular characteristics of the quality of spermatozoa or with the method of insemination. As noted in Section 6 above, valid evaluation of such correlations and of the merits of AIH itself in cases of questionable semen quality is both complicated and limited, even with the better-designed investigations.

8. APPLICATIONS OF CRYOBANKING IN AIH

Cryobanking should be as feasible and as effective for husband semen in AIH as it is for donor semen in AID, provided that the potentially fertile spermatozoa show a cryosurvival preferably of at least 50% in terms of progressive motility. The degree of cryosurvival cannot be predicted on the basis of population density, motility, abnormal forms, or even fertility of spermatozoa in semen, since there are no established correlations of these, or any such factors, with sensitivity to freezing and thawing. This precludes selection of ejaculates for cryobanking without first screening for survival during freezing and thawing. This is true not only in ejaculates from different individuals, but also from ejaculates of the same individual, because physical as well as physiological characteristics may change between collections. In general, however, good-quality semen is more likely to favor preservation by freezing than specimens showing oligospermia with related asthenospermia and a high percentage of abnormal forms, but good-quality semen may or may not show good cryo-survival.

Cryobanking of husband's semen has introduced four distinct clinical applications which are not possible with fresh semen, in addition to extending the potential and actual advantages of AIH with fresh semen (see Sections 1 and 4 above).

8.1. Pre-vasectomy storage

Semen can be frozen and stored prior to vasectomy to favor the maintenance of fertility potential subsequent to surgically induced sterility, in the event children are desired at a later date because of tragic loss, changes in family planning or marital status, and so on. The early expectation that a significant number of the projected 750,000 men seeking sterilization each year would choose pre-vasectomy storage has not developed at all (Sherman 1973, 1977). It is surprising that the vast majority of men seem indifferent to the advantages of cryobanking in maintaining their fertility potential. Most are reluctant to undergo the inconvenience involved, especially the required abstinence period between each of the three to five collections (ejaculations) needed to provide enough semen for processing a reasonable number of insemination units (about 0.5 ml per unit) for use in AIH on demand in subsequent attempts to effect fertilization. The practice, however, is still viable and shows signs of slow but consistent growth, even in the face of improved surgical procedures for reversal of functional as well as structural effects of vasectomy. Efficacy of cryopreservation and fertility expectation should be the same as that expected for donor cryobanking in AID provided semen quality is comparable.

8.2. Pre-therapy storage

This category concerns cryopreservation of semen prior to radiotherapy and/or chemotherapy as well as certain surgical procedures to offset the possible danger of these treatments in causing sterility or possible adverse mutagenic consequences in aberrant spermatogenesis or early development. In contrast to pre-vasectomy storage, there is a recent and more active awareness of the role of cryobanking prior to the possibility of deleterious exposure of men to either surgical or non-surgical therapy, especially for cancer, which may compromise the integrity of the reproductive process. The author has received an increased number of inquiries and requests for consultations concerning appropriate cryo-banking facilities in various geographic locations throughout the United States, some involving the desire of hospitals or clinics to establish their own banks exclusively for pre-therapy storage. I look for much greater clinical use of cryobanking in this area of application in AIH, especially in institutions which specialize in cancer therapy. Research efforts should parallel this clinical activity, directed at providing more information on the potential deleterious effects of such treatments on spermatozoa in physical and genetic development. Such research could and should very easily and rationally parallel the practical appli-cation of cryobanks used with such patients. A limitation in application, at least, in some conditions of malignancy, may be the reduction of semen quality in the course of the disease itself. If initially recognized as a possibility, the advantage of cryopreservation of semen early on after the detection of disease is strongly recommended. Given semen of average characteristics of quality, there is reason to expect fertility results comparable with those realized with AID.

8.3. Storage in retrograde ejaculation

Semen from retrograde ejaculation has been recovered from the bladder, cryo-preserved for clinical use and used successfully in AIH (Dmowski et al., this volume, charter 13). The clinical advantage of storage of such specimens in cases of irregular and unpredictable ovulation is obvious. However, even if the wife has normal cycles, cryobanking will allow storage of part of the semen specimen for future use. This will minimize the attendant risk associated with a need for repeated catheterizations to procure semen for AIH.

8.4. Storage in oligospermia

The majority of male factor infertility cases are thought to be due to poor-quality semen with obvious oligospermia, asthenospermia and often an associated high percentage of abnormal forms. The actual causes of male infertility due to semen may be numerous, undetected, unexplained and for the most part incapable of correction. The factors which are described in the collective term 'quality of semen (spermatozoa)' are critical to the integrity of both fertilization and early embryogenesis. The frequent cryosensitivity of poor-quality semen (Colton and Farris 1958; Rubin et al. 1969; Sherman 1964) presents a serious limitation in the use of cryobanking to enhance indications for AIH in infertility therapy which is associated with semen quality (Sherman 1973). Even if cryosurvival is optimal for poor-quality spermatozoa, frozen storage alone cannot be expected a priori to correct the deficiencies in these factors.

The desperation of infertile couples, whose difficulty is attributed to husband's oligospermia, perhaps makes them look upon cryobanking with AIH as the only personal or private solution to their problem. This application of cryobanking, unfortunately, is the least likely to produce a pregnancy. The procedure, nevertheless, should be considered as the final step in AIH before resorting to AID or adoption. It should be recommended and utilized with a degree of pessimism, however, even after careful evaluation of the male as to suitability of his semen for cryobanking and reasonable recovery of a sufficient number of normal motile cells for insemination.

Many ejaculates from oligospermic husbands can be collected, frozen and stored over a period of weeks or months, thawed, pooled, concentrated by mild centrifugation and then inseminated at spermatozoal concentrations manifoldly greater than the original single ejaculates (Sherman 1964) or than the superior portions of split ejaculates. The concentration of single ejaculates can also precede frozen storage if desired. This technique can be expected to achieve success, in principle, when used in cases where a deficiency in number of motile spermatozoa is the only cause of male infertility. It is more probable, however, that factors of infertility other than reduced numbers of spermatozoa are involved with the oligospermia, and that successful application of cryobanking in its 'treatment', therefore, is quite limited because it increases the number without improving the quality of spermatozoa. In addition, oligospermic samples usually show a poor recovery after freezing and thawing as they are more sensitive to cryoinjury (Sherman 1964). This further restricts the application of this procedure in clinical practice. The general steps recommended for the procedure are:

A. Establishment of the suitability of semen on the basis of complete semen analysis of three ejaculates, each preceded by 3 to 5 days of abstinence, with appropriate minimum or standard values for spermatozoa of above 5 million/cc density, fair to good quality of motility, above 45% progressive motility, below 30% abnormalities of head and neck, and cryosurvival of above 40%, as well as at least 2 ml for semen volume;

B. Collection of about 10 or more ejaculates for each concentrated insemination unit, the number being dependent on the data provided in the initial semen analysis of each ejaculate. The aim is to deliver at least 50 million normal-appearing, motile spermatozoa in each insemination – the spermatozoa from these ejaculates may be concentrated and then frozen or frozen as they are for subsequent concentration after thawing;

C. Freezing of semen in plastic straws or glass ampules in 0.5-1.0 ml aliquots, as appropriate, in liquid nitrogen vapor ($-190°$ to $-196°$C), or in air at $-80°$ to $-85°$C, and subsequent storage under liquid nitrogen ($-196°$C) – details of cryopreservation techniques are presented under Section 12;

D. Just prior to insemination, the number of frozen samples required to satisfy the delivery of at least 50 million progressively motile, normal-appearing spermatozoa are thawed and pooled into one sample;

E. The pooled sample then is centrifuged in a conical tube at about 4,000 rpm for about 5 minutes and all but a volume of 0.2 to 1 ml is discarded – the volume is determined by the mode of insemination;

F. The centrifugate or plug of spermatozoa then is mixed gently by pipette action with the supernatant above it, and the pooled concentrate of 0.2 to 1 ml in the preparation is inseminated.

9. SPECIAL TREATMENT OF EJACULATES

In spite of the slim chances for success, increasing numbers of infertile couples who are faced with obvious oligospermia will elect to use cryobanking with AIH as a last resort to realizing fatherhood by the husband. Patients should be cautioned as to the pessimistic outlook of the procedure for the reasons discussed above and discouraged from its pursuit, especially if semen evaluation is far below reasonable standards. The degree of success of this treatment may be a very lów percentage in relative terms of patient numbers, but it is actually 100% in terms of happiness and fulfillment for those fortunate, successful patients. Cryobanking for concentration of spermatozoa, therefore, should be available for current use, but its techniques must be improved if it is to play an important role in male infertility therapy.

The future effectiveness of cryobanking in AIH with poor-quality ejaculates obviously depends upon special treatment of spermatozoa in vitro to increase their fertility potential somehow by changing their characteristics in a population. Improvement in cryosurvival, no doubt, will play an important role in the effectiveness of cryobanking for AIH, but only when the spermatozoa preserved by better techniques in vitro are capable of fertilization after their insemination.

9.1. Split ejaculate technique

The recognition that AIH of whole ejaculates alone may not compensate for the infertility factor of deficiency in number of progressively moving spermatozoa in the ejaculate suggested the concentration of spermatozoa in semen before its use. The concept of a physiological concentration by obtaining the best portion of a partitioned or split ejaculate was introduced (Shields 1950, Farris and Murphy 1960), probably to avoid the inconvenience, questionable rationale, and possible deleterious alterations of in vitro handling during concentration by centrifugation and resuspension. The. split ejaculate technique favors the collection of that portion of the ejaculate, almost always the first, which contains the highest density of the most active and progressively motile, normal-appearing spermatozoa (Amelar and Hotchkiss 1965). Not all investigators, however, are in total agreement with this popular doctrine (Eliasson and Lindholmer 1972). The practiced assumption, nevertheless, is that the portion with the spermatozoal population of highest density is more capable of effecting fertilization than either the other portion or the whole ejaculate. The technique is advocated or suggested by the experiences of some practitioners as a favorable clinical measure in the treatment of infertility with AIH (Finegold 1976; Moghissi et al. 1977; Dixon et al. 1976; Ulstein 1973; Steiman and Taymor 1977; Barwin 1974).

If, indeed, the use of the split ejaculate technique in AIH increases the percentage of fertility of subfertile couples, then it follows that cryobanking should further increase the chances of AIH for successful pregnancy. Superior split ejaculate semen samples could be preserved by freezing for subsequent use at times most appropriate for AIH in single or multiple inseminations during the female cycle. In addition, such samples could be concentrated in vitro either before or after frozen storage to enhance further the principle of delivery to the female tract of as many good-quality spermatozoa as possible. This principle has been demonstrated successfully in limited but growing clinical practice in Austria by Gasser et al. (1978), and in the United States by Keswani and Clitheroe (1978). These experts in infertility therapy further concentrated, by centrifugation, the most concentrated portions of split parts of oligospermic ejaculates which were then preserved by freezing until needed for AIH. This application of cryobanking in AIH has resulted in 11 pregnancies, 5 of which have already come to normal term (Table 1). However, both investigators complicated evaluation of their results by adding fresh semen of the husband to

Table 1. Recent results of AIH with cryopreserved semen in cases of oligospermia.

Investigator	No. of cases	No. of preg- nancies	No. of abor- tions	No. of births	Percent preg- nancies
Barkay et al. (1977): Israel	32	15*	2	9	47
Barwin (1974): Ireland (31)	20	11	4	***	55
Decker (1978): United States	155	27**	4	17	18
Gasser et al (1978): Austria	63	6	***	***	10
Keswani and Clitheroe (1978): United State	31	5	0	5	16
Nakamura (1978): Brazil	100	16	5	11	16
Sillo-Seidl (1972): Germany	12	8	2	6	67

   * Four current
  ** Six current
*** No data available

each cryopreserved specimen just before insemination. Such a practice compromises absolute assignment of fertilizing capacity to the frozen-stored spermatozoa. The previous long-term history of male infertility in these patients, however, makes this assignment most probable if not definite.

9.2. Intrauterine insemination

Success in insemination obviously depends upon the functional integrity of the gametes and reproductive systems, as well as proper timing as to ovulation. In addition, chances for pregnancy with AIH, especially in cases of male factor infertility, may be markedly improved by the method of insemination employed. It is advantageous to insure that as many spermatozoa as possible are placed in the most favorable environment for their transport to the site of fertilization. In principle, intrauterine insemination appears to satisfy this requirement under certain conditions associated with causative factors in infertility.

The chemical and/or physical environment of the vagina, cervix and cervical mucus is sometimes hostile to spermatozoa in semen, preventing their proper deposition and transport for fertilization. Intrauterine insemination has been used to bypass these structures in infertility therapy (Parish and Ward 1968). Its use in AIH, in principle, seems logical but here as with other factors considered in the evaluation of AIH, there are differences of opinion and clinical practices as to suitability, success and safety. Postcoital examinations or cervical mucus tests for the presence, motility, penetration and agglutination status of spermatozoa have served as indicators of a favorable or unfavorable environment for potential success in reproduction.

Guttmacher (1960) doubted the efficacy of intrauterine insemination and recommended estrogen treatment instead. He considered it justified only in cases of cervical catarrh secondary to local infection or when a pinpoint external os prevents passage and deposition of cervical mucus. Mastroianni et al. (1957) compared the various methods of insemination and, in terms of rate of success in AIH and possible adverse side effects, felt that the use of the intrauterine route should be abandoned. Kleegman and Kaufman (1966) reported that among infertile couples with male factor infertility based upon poor semen quality, the extent of success with intrauterine insemination was a pregnancy rate of 20%. But among the failures in this series with AIH who continued with normal coitus, the subsequent pregnancy rate was even higher. The efficacy of AIH even with intrauterine insemination, therefore, was questioned by these workers. Intrauterine insemination in AIH, however, was recommended by Kleegman and Kaufman (1966) in cases of poor postcoital tests, especially using the split ejaculate, but only to physicians who have expert knowledge of indications, contraindications and technique. Cohen (1962) advocates this type of insemination as efficacious and safe. Intrauterine insemination was compared with other techniques and found to produce the highest pregnancy rate in AIH (Kaskarelis and Comminos 1959). Recently, Ulstein (1973) realized about 33% success with the intrauterine method in AIH for infertility therapy, reporting also that the in vitro test for sperm penetration of cervical mucus was the best index of fertility potential in its positive correlation with semen quality. It has been reported also that fewer progressively motile spermatozoa are required in achieving pregnancy with intrauterine insemination than with other techniques (Sillo-Seidl 1978). Barwin (1974) reported unbelievable success with AIH of cryopreserved semen using intrauterine insemination in cases of male infertility, including oligospermia (Table 1). He concluded that intrauterine insemination of husband's semen has a definite place in the treatment of infertility.

Intrauterine insemination also may be valuable in delivering directly to the uterine cavity the required small volume of semen (no more than 0.5 ml) with a more concentrated population of the highest-quality spermatozoa which is obtained from initially poor-quality ejaculates appropriately treated in vitro. This is suggested by recent success in fertility resulting from insemination of spermatozoa isolated from filtered semen (Dmowski et al. 1978; Black et al. 1978). This suggestion is made in spite of the claim by some experienced practitioners that with poor-quality semen results will be unsatisfactory regardless of the method of insemination (Guttmacher 1960; Kleegman and Kaufman 1966).

9.3. In vitro treatment of spermatozoa

AIH has the potential to become an important therapeutic tool in infertility when semen quality is poor. It permits a variety of in vitro treatments of deficient semen, in addition to cell concentration by centrifugation, which are designed to improve the fertilizing capacity of its spermatozoa. AIH also insures, by selection of an appropriate method, the deposition of treated or untreated spermatozoa at that site in the female reproductive tract which is considered optimal to effect fertilization. If in vitro methods for increasing reproductive capacity are devised which could be further enhanced by selective AIH, then the chief cause of male infertility will be minimized, or even obviated.

Early attempts at in vitro treatment of human semen involved the substitution of various diluents for seminal plasma, after its removal by centrifugation, to revive or stimulate motility of spermatozoa (Granzow 1932; Hirakawa 1909; Mettenleiter 1925). There were no reports of pregnancies after insemination of such substituted semen. Rosin (1958), however, reported pregnancies following the use of seminal plasma from a donor as the substitute fluid. Eckerling (1960) demonstrated that increased motility and subsequent pregnancies resulted from the use of human blood serum as the vehicle for spermatozoa in seminal plasma-substituted ejaculates of infertile husbands. Current accepted procedures in AIH, however, do not ordinarily include such methods in accepted and efficacious practice.

Schoenfeld et al. (1975) showed that the addition of caffeine to semen in vitro increased not only the percentage motility but also the forward progression and lifespan of spermatozoa, especially in poor-quality ejaculates. They proposed the clinical use of caffeine with poor-quality semen prior to AIH to improve its fertilizing capacity. Recently, Harrison (1978) completed a study in which results of AIH were compared using semen with and without the addition of caffeine. In spite of the enhanced motility of spermatozoa inseminated, no pregnancies occurred with the caffeine-stimulated semen with either normal or subnormal-quality spermatozoa. The addition of caffeine to human semen, therefore, was discouraged by this author whose data also suggested that caffeine may damage spermatozoa in some way. It is known that caffeine may alter chromosomes (Kihlman 1977), which means that it could possibly function as a mutagenic agent in such applications.

Barkay et al. (1977) found that caffeine increases the motility of cryopreserved spermatozoa when it is added to semen either before freezing or during thawing. Caffeine stimulation appeared greater, however, with the poorer samples which showed both asthenospermia and oligospermia. Barkay and his associates (personal communication, 1978) have carried this observation further into clinical practice of both AIH and AID for infertility therapy. Results of insemination with frozen-stored semen in 1974-1976 without caffeine were compared with results of 1976-1978 with caffeine (Table 2). Although the number of cases is not large, 114 for AID and 32 for AIH, there was a 10% increase in the pregnancy rate which resulted from caffeine treatment of semen in both groups. Barkay's group has therefore established that caffeine in either donor or husband semen is compatible with the fertilization and the development of apparently normal progeny. The abortion rate in the caffeine series was actually below normal, occurring in only 5 out of 90 pregnancies, or 5.5%. There is no evidence, at least from these data, therefore, that caffeine is harmful or mutagenic to spermatozoa.

Table 2. Effect of caffeine on fertilizing capacity of cryopreserved spermatozoa in AIH and AID (from Barkay et al. 1977).

Treatment (period)	Insemination	No. of cases	No. of births	No. of spontaneous abortions	No. of current pregnancies	Total pregnancies	% pregnancies
Without	AID	46	18	2	7	27	59
caffeine	AIH	10	1	1	2	4	40
(1974-76)							
Total		56	19	3	9	31	55
With	AID	68	37	4	6	47	69
caffeine	AIH	22	8	1	2	11	50
(1976-78)							
Total		90	45	5	8	58	64

There is another substance, hog pancreatic kallikrein, which has been used successfully, in oral administration, to increase the number of spermatozoa as well as the percentage and quality of motility in subfertile men. In a double-blind study, pregnancy rates induced by kallikrein-treated patients were more than twice those of the placebo group (Schill 1977). In vitro treatment was also shown to improve the extent and quality of spermatozoal motility in semen samples which initially showed reduced motility, as well as in semen samples which had been cryopreserved. Schill proposed the use of kallikrein in combination with AIH as a therapeutic measure designed to improve cervical mucus penetration and favor fertilization in appropriate cases of infertility. If this proves success-ful, then its clinical use in AIH would be enhanced with the on-demand storage advantages of cryobanking.

9.4. Isolation and separation of spermatozoa

Centrifugation has been used for some time to increase the population density of spermatozoa within an ejaculate for use in AIH, in attempts to offset original oligospermia (Hansen and Rock 1951). Pooling and concentration of a number of ejaculates preserved by freezing may be employed to increase the efficiency of such concentration greatly. Chances of marked success in effecting fertility, however, are remote even with cryobanking because of other deficiencies in quality of spermatozoa which are not corrected by concentration alone (Sherman 1973). Complete isolation of spermatozoa from seminal plasma, in-cluding antibodies associated with their immobilization and their agglutina-tion, can be accomplished by filtration of semen through millipore filters (Jecht and Poon 1975). This technique may provide a means of treating ejaculates prior to AIH in cases of infertility due to antibodies which, if present, could prevent fertilization. Plasma-free spermatozoa would, of course, be resuspended in suitable physiological fluids or even spermatozoa-free seminal plasma of appropriate donor semen which is prepared by millipore filtration prior to insemination.

Ericsson (1977) reported on a method of filtering human semen through a column of serum albumin which isolates most of the progressively motile sper-matozoa from the constituents of seminal plasma as well as from immotile, poorly motile, and structurally abnormal spermatozoa, but with considerable loss in cell numbers. Such isolated, highly motile spermatozoa also demonstrated improved cryosurvival after storage at $-196°$ C compared with split-sample unfiltered specimens. The application of this method with AIH, either with single small samples of fresh semen or with pooled and concentrated multiple samples of frozen-stored ejaculates, could increase in conception rate in infertility therapy. In an initial clinical trial, spermatozoa were isolated from fresh semen of infertile husbands for use in intrauterine AIH (Glass and Ericsson 1978). None of the 19 patients inseminated became pregnant however. The authors suggested that pregnancy failure might be due to the intrinsic inability to fertilize of even the best spermatozoa isolated from a poor-quality sample. More recent clinical application of this method, however, has resulted in 12 births and 6 current pregnancies (Black et al. 1978; Dmowski et al. 1978; Ericsson, personal communication, 1978). It should be recognized that the concept of improved fertility with a 'clean' population of spermatozoa, 'free' from cells of poor motility and abnormal structure as well as debris of the plasma, has not been established by these results. Well-designed comparative studies with larger numbers of cases are required, but the outlook is encouraging, with exciting possibilities especially in the relationship of the isolation technique to AIH with cryobanked semen from subfertile husbands.

10. SEMEN QUALITY IN AIH AND ABNORMALITIES OF PREGNANCY

Pregnancy is of little beneficial consequence to the potential and aim of the reproductive process in general and of AIH in particular, unless it is completed with the birth of a normal child. Spontaneous abortion is a salient obstacle to such progeny development. It has been proposed that spermatozoa may be a factor in interrupting normal pregnancy; but the defined role of subnormal quality of spermatozoa, expressed as increased abnormal forms and reduced motility, in the induction of spontaneous abortion, is controversial. The clinical experience of Kleegman and Kaufman (1966) reveals that the rate of spontaneous abortion increases with the use of poor-quality semen which initially is successful in insemination by achieving pregnancy. A high number of spontaneous abortions, 11 of 46 cases in AIH, or 24%, also suggested a relationship with oligospermia (with asthenospermia) to Sillo-Seidl in his report (personal communication, 1978). Data were not presented, however, concerning the reasonable expectation that a higher percentage of abnormally formed spermatozoa was associated with the oligospermia he observed (Moghissi et al. 1977). Recent results with AIH, not noted as such by the authors but seen in their published data, show high abortion rates of 32% (Usherwood et al. 1976) and 60% (Ulstein 1973) after fertilization with oligospermic and asthenospermic semen specimens. Moghissi et al. (1977) discussed their subsequent findings of considerable pregnancy wastage after initially realizing good pregnancy rates with AIH, suggesting its relationship with the high proportion of structural abnormalities in populations of spermatozoa used. Thiede, however, in discussing the paper by Moghissi et al. (1977), points out that it is difficult to ascribe a level of significance to speculations concerning any relationship between abnormal spermatozoa and pregnancy wastage because of inadequate controls and design of investigations.

In an extensive study MacLeod and Gold (1957) found no correlation between either structure of spermatozoa specifically or quality of semen in general, and any type of failure in pregnancy. Other authors have reached the same conclusion (Bender 1952; Swyer 1953; Russell 1954; Joel 1955; Hartman 1946). There is data also that in a large series of cases involving accidents of pregnancy, the quality of semen inseminated was superior, not inferior (MacLeod and Gold 1957). A recent report by Glass and Golbus (1978) stated that 'the role, if any, of the male in habitual abortion is unknown .

The uncertain nature of the relationship discussed opens to question the rationale and validity of attempts at improving clinical success of AIH in infertility therapy by removing abnormal spermatozoa from the insemination unit. Such removal of many to most abnormal forms is now possible with recently introduced filtration or isolation techniques (Ericsson 1977; Glass and Golbus 1978). It is considered one of the advantages of these methods in infertility therapy with AIH, along with separation of the spermatozoa on the basis of sex and progressive motility, which they are proposed to effect. Recent advances in cytogenetics strongly implicate intrinsic defects (chromosomal aberrations) in the zygote as the most likely cause of abnormal development and fetal wastage, not the structural form of the gametes (Fabricant et al. 1978). This makes the positive relationship between abnormal-appearing spermatozoa and spontaneous abortion unlikely rather than uncertain.

11. RESULTS WITH CRYOBANKING IN AIH

The first successful use of cryobanking with AIH resulted in the birth of a beautiful baby girl (Sherman et al., unpublished observations, 1954). Multiple samples of frozen-stored oligospermic semen were thawed, pooled and concentrated by centrifugation before insemination. There were two other successful applications with concentration, cryobanking and AIH reported (Sawada 1964; Behrman and Sawada 1966).

A total of only 16 births from cryopreserved husband semen was reported as a statistic by Sherman (1976), but no details as to the application, methods or semen characteristics were available for tabulation. It was Sillo-Seidl (1972), however, who first published documentation of details of semen characteristics, treatment, pregnancies and births following cryobanking for concentration in AIH. He introduced the use of the term 'fertility index' (volume × cell density × % progressively moving, normal-appearing spermatozoa) which emphasized the importance of progressively motile spermatozoa with normal structure as the key ingredient in achieving pregnancy. A fertility index of 50 million was suggested and used clinically by him for successful application in eight out of twelve cases of frozen storage with concentration of semen in AIH. This use of cryobanking in oligospermia relative to its dramatic potential in principle, however, has been a disappointment in practice. Certainly it has proven to be less than spectacular in clinical application (Behrman 1975). Ledward et al. (1977) suggested that the method is unsuitable in the management of the oligospermic males after no pregnancies in AIH were obtained in 10 cases. They also observed no pregnancies, however, after cell concentration and use of fresh semen in AIH.

There has been relatively little activity in AIH with frozen-stored semen compared to that in AID according to current available information. The very incomplete, essentially token feedback from questionnaires and personal contacts, as well as from a few publications and pre-publication manuscripts, reveals a total of only 88 recent pregnancies and 48 births to date from cryopreserved semen used for infertility associated with oligospermia. The average percentage of spontaneous abortions, as with cryopreserved semen used in AID, appears below that of the normal population in this small series, although there is variation between investigators. No abnormalities of birth have been reported (Table 1). Most of these successes have been realized through the preliminary use of in vitro treatments or techniques, the use of which was suggested first by improvement of poor-quality semen from ejaculates used in AIH with fresh semen (see Section 9).

There is no published summary of data on the number of pregnancies and births resulting from the use of cryobanked semen in AIH in specifically identified applications other than oligospermia (Table 1). Two normal births were reported, however, with pre-vasectomy husband semen stored for over two years in Arkansas, and one normal birth after six years of frozen storage for the same purpose in Minnesota (Sherman, Olson, personal observations, 1978). These three cases, all successful, apparently are the only ones attempted with pre-vasectomy semen stored in these two cryobanks and suggest the expected favorable potential of this application. In each case, semen was from fertile husbands whose fertility was maintained in a cryobank. It is likely that some of the 16 births reported (Sherman 1976) included both oligospermic and pre-vasectomy semen, but responses to questionnaires did not identify the application in AIH. It is likely that a number of pregnancies and births have resulted from cryopreserved semen in AIH in various applications, but they are unreported and unknown. Readers are invited to send such reports to me or to the Reproductive Council of AATB (12111 Parklawn Drive, Rockville, Maryland 20852, USA).

Encouragement for realizing the potential of other applications is given in recent success with the use of cryopreserved semen preserved and used in AIH therapy for infertility after retrograde ejaculation (Kapetanakis et al. 1978; Dmowski et al., this volume, Chapter 13) and in case of a paraplegic husband (Chapelle et al. 1976).

There is a possibility that if a factor in male infertility is due to antibodies carried on the surface of spermatozoa, cryobanking in AIH will reduce its deleterious role. It has been suggested recently that freezing and thawing reduces the antigenicity of human spermatozoa (Alexander and Kay 1977).

Nakamura and his associates during the past ten years in Brazil have had considerable experience in AIH with fresh and more recently with cryopreserved semen. Details as to likely and established causes of infertility, especially as to degree of oligospermia, have been documented in one of the most complete studies with a relatively large number of cases (Nakamura 1978; Nakamura and Ramos 1975).

12. TECHNIQUES IN CRYOBANKING

The principles and practices of current techniques used in cryopreservation of human semen were presented recently (Sherman 1977). I was asked by the editors to repeat the schematic summary of my recommended liquid nitrogen vapor method in this chapter. The reader is referred to the original source for details, photographs of equipment, and for discussion of the pellet-freezing method. Nakamura and Ramos (1975) use the classic simple pellet-freezing method with solid carbon dioxide (dry ice) in Brazil (Nagase and Niwa 1974), while a semi-automatic, electronically-controlled liquid-nitrogen freezing apparatus for pellets (Figure 1) is used in Israel by Barkay (personal communication, 1978). Both experts in infertility extend semen with an egg-yolk diluter and have had success in AIH with cryopreserved pellets of oligospermic specimens (Table 1, Figure 1).

The following methods, which the author has found suitable for the preservation of many types of cells, can be instituted easily, inexpensively and successfully in the establishment of a modest clinical bank in a hospital laboratory or even in a physician's office. Unless otherwise specified, all steps or treatments which follow are conducted at room temperature ($\pm$ 22° C). Figure 2 depicts these steps in cryopreservation and the equipment used.

I. *Semen is collected* after a three-to-five-day abstinence period, by masturbation into a sterile 2-oz glass or polypropylene wide-mouthed ointment jar. The abstinence period favors a degree of both standardization and assurance of a superior population of progressively moving cells. Liquid semen is ejaculated but it immediately coagulates into a gel.

II. When the *coagulated semen* liquefies, usually within 30 minutes, its volume is measured by drawing it up into a 5-ml syringe with an 18-gauge needle. It is then returned to the jar or to a 10-ml. Erlenmeyer flask. A small aliquot ($\pm$ 0.2 ml) is usually removed for a semen analysis (percentage, type and duration of motility, viability staining, cell density, abnormalities, and the like).

III. *Glycerol* is added to semen with a medicine dropper in a stepwise fashion,

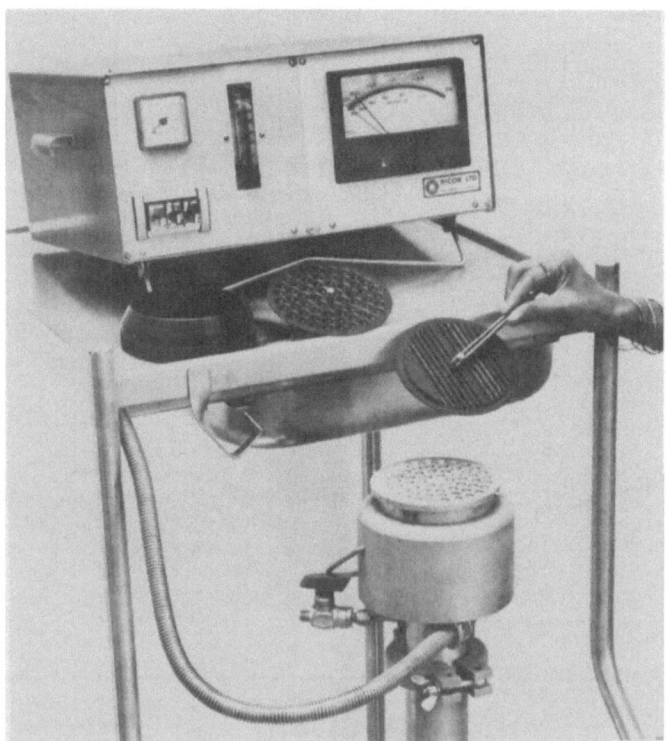

Figure 1. Electronic semi-automatic system for pellet freezing. Human semen, diluted 1:1 with egg-yolk citrate, glycerol and antibiotics. is frozen as 0.15 ml pellets in non-stick depressions in a metal plate cooled by controlled flow of liquid nitrogen. Pellets are transferred with a plastic spoon to test tube containing liquid nitrogen; the test tube is stoppered with gauze and transferred to liquid-nitrogen storage refrigerator. When semen is needed for insemination, test tube is removed with forceps and about seven pellets are placed in a dry eprouvette for thawing in a bath at +37° C. Reprinted from Sherman (1977) with permission of Elsevier North-Holland Press, Amsterdam.

one drop per 10-14 drops of semen, figuring 20 drops per ml of semen volume. The jar or flask is swirled gently after each addition for mixing. One minute is allowed between additions. A final concentration of about 7-10% by volume is satisfactory. Exact quantitation, therefore, is unnecessary, but volumetric step-wise additions can be made, if preferred, on the basis of the percentage glycerol by volume desired. If an extender such as egg-yolk citrate is used, semen is diluted 1:1 by stepwise additions of the extender with twice the glycerol concentration required in the final mixture. Recent experiments in our laboratory reveal no difference between 5, 7.5 and 10% glycerol in the cryoprotection of undiluted (raw) semen on the basis of progressive motility.

IV. *Glycerolated semen* is then placed into plastic straws (paillettes) or glass ampules for subsequent freezing and storage or, if preferred, the treated semen is frozen outside of a container, as pellets.

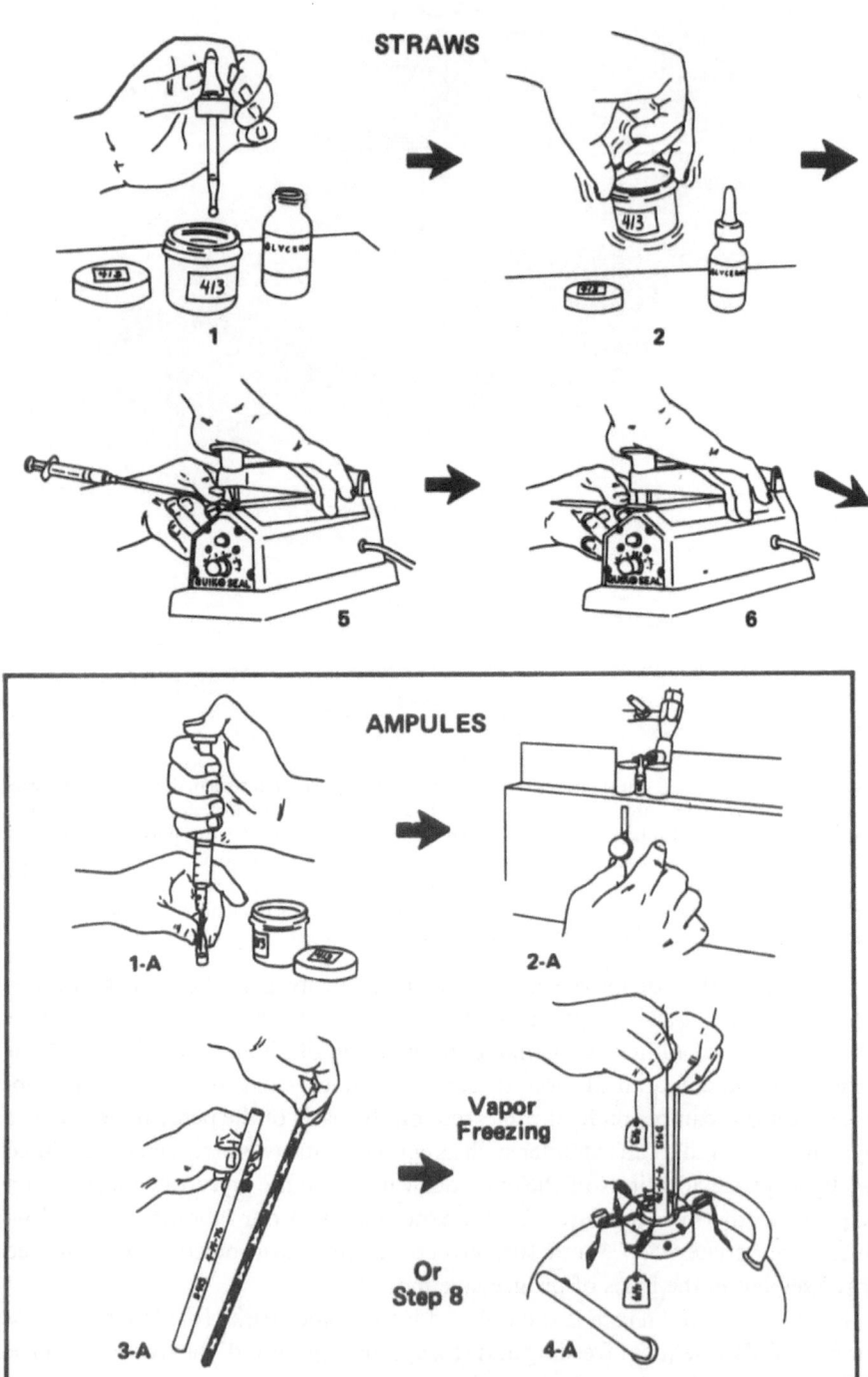

STRAWS

1

2

5

6

AMPULES

1-A

2-A

3-A

Vapor
Freezing

Or
Step 8

4-A

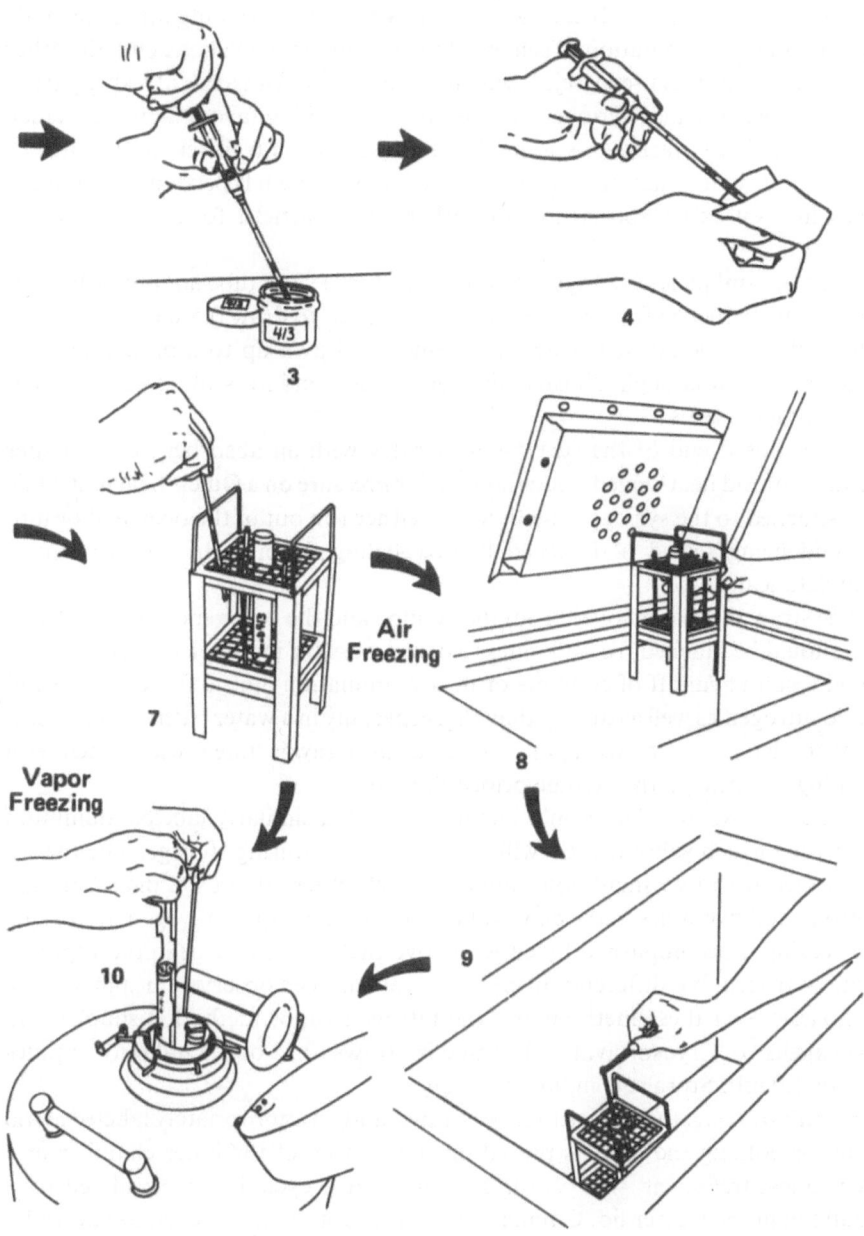

Figure 2. Schematic representation of the major steps in freezing human semen in plastic straws and glass ampules in refrigerated air ($-85°$ C) and in liquid nitrogen vapor ($-190°$ to $-196°$ C), with storage in liquid nitrogen ($-196°$ C). Reprinted from Sherman (1977) with permission of North-Holland Press, Amsterdam.

A. *Straws*. Straws (0.5 ml) used are one of two types, depending upon the mode of subsequent insemination of semen. One has a nylon plug at one end; the other does not. The plug is used to eject semen when pushed with a metal rod as part of a special insemination syringe. The absence of the plug favors a greater semen capacity and may facilitate sealing, but requires semen transfer to a syringe or cup in another insemination technique. A Sharpie fine felt pen with permanent black ink is used to label straws and other related articles for identification in storage.

A 2.5 or 5-ml plastic syringe, fitted with a short Tygon tube adaptor (about 3-mm inside diameter) for holding the straw, is used to draw 0.5-0.6 ml of semen into each suitable labeled straw. The semen is drawn up to a premarked line which will allow enough adjusted air space at each end for sealing without fluid contacting the seals.

The exposed end of the straw is wiped dry with an absorbent tissue paper (Kimwipe) and heat-sealed electrically under pressure on a Quick-Seal unit while still attached to the syringe. The fluid will either run out of the open end or into the end being sealed if detached before sealing. Wiping dry helps insure a complete seal.

The straw then is removed from the syringe and the other end is sealed. Each seal should be pinched from its sides to detect possible incomplete sealing which could result in runoff of contents or in contamination during frozen storage in liquid nitrogen as well as during thawing, especially in a water bath. Reseal if seal is incomplete. If straws with plugs are used, the straw is 'filled' with semen with the plug end next to the syringe prior to sealing.

Sealed straws are placed on a metal rack with a similarly labeled aluminum cigar tube which subsequently will hold the straws during storage. The tube is perforated with two small holes opposite each other, about 3/8 inch from the bottom, and two holes in the cap to allow entrance of liquid nitrogen in storage.

Freezing is accomplished by either of two methods, in air or in the vapor of liquid nitrogen. No difference in cryosurvival has been observed in split-sample comparisons of these methods but the nitrogen vapor method is simpler and less expensive. Cryosurvival is the same in straws (0.25 or 0.5 ml) and ampules (0.5 or 1.0 ml). Storage is in liquid nitrogen.

For *air freezing*, the rack with tube, straws, and an appropriately labeled metal cane for holding the tube, is placed on the bottom of the inner chamber of a mechanical freezer at $-85°$ C for a 10-30-minute cycle in air circulated by a small fan in the freezer lid. Circulation of air is optional, however, as shown by recent studies. The actual length of the cycle depends upon freezing rate and convenience of laboratory operation, but the semen reaches $-80°C$ in about 10 minutes.

After the freezing cycle, straws are quickly placed in the tube by grasping their top seals with forceps. The tube is closed with its metal screw-type cap.

The tube is snapped on to the labeled metal cane with gloved hand and then quickly transferred into a labeled canister in a neighbouring 30-liter liquid-nitrogen storage refrigerator. The transfer of the straws to the tube and then to the refrigerator is performed in haste within the mechanical freezer to prevent undue warm-up.

The canister is quickly lowered into the liquid nitrogen for frozen storage. The liquid nitrogen surrounds the tubes and the straws within since both canister and tubes are perforated. If the tube is to be added to a cane already in storage, the rapid transfer is made to the cane lifted momentarily from the canister. Each cane has a capacity for holding two tubes. If such operations are more complicated, transfers and rearrangements should be made via a separate liquid nitrogen bath, to minimize warm-up of stored material.

In *liquid nitrogen vapor freezing*, sealed straws are placed in the cigar tube which is closed with its screw cap and placed in a metal cane at room temperature.

The cane with tube is then placed into a liquid-nitrogen-tight canister which is raised for this transfer from its seated position in a liquid-nitrogen refrigerator. The special nitrogen-tight canister is prepared from the standard one by sealing the side seam with silver solder and closing its perforated bottom with a metal plug. A brass plug 1/4-1/2-inch thick provides the necessary weight to prevent floating in liquid nitrogen.

The canister is quickly lowered and reseated in the refrigerator whose liquid-nitrogen level is just below that of the open top of the canister, permitting only vapor contact with specimens to be frozen. The freezing rate achieved with vapor freezing, not the much more rapid rate with liquid freezing, is more favorable to preservation.

After 30 minutes or when convenient during the work day, the cane is transferred to a standard canister with a perforated bottom for storage in liquid nitrogen – not in its vapor – either in the same or another refrigerator.

Proper storage requires maintenance of temperatures at or near −196° C. Nitrogen levels should always be maintained accordingly. Handling of specimens outside the container in bright light should be minimized. A log with weekly recorded checks on levels with a wooden yardstick is recommended. The frost-line measurement after immersion is a simple, accurate guide to filling. Pressure filling from another 30-liter refrigerator is recommended and most economical.

B. *Ampules*. Labeled, prescored glass ampules of 0.5 or 1-ml capacity, are filled by transfer from a 5-ml hypodermic syringe with an 18-gauge needle. Care is taken to avoid touching the wet needle to the tip in withdrawing to prevent 'burn' and internal smoking during sealing. Slight negative pressure keeps semen within the needle during withdrawal. The needle is wiped before filling for the same reason.

Ampules are tip-sealed by flame in a semi-automatic pharmaceutical machine and snapped on labeled metal canes.

Each cane is placed in a labeled cardboard sleeve and this assembly is transferred to a weighted and sealed liquid-nitrogen-tight canister for freezing and frozen storage in the vapor of liquid nitrogen, as described above for straws. Canes can be frozen without sleeves with the same cryosurvival, if preferred.

Ampules on metal canes with or without cardboard sleeves also can be frozen and stored in the mechanical freezer (-85°C) bij standing them upright, inserted at their bottom ends in a styrafoam base. After 30 minutes, canes are placed in the cooled sleeves in the freezer and quickly transferred to a standard perforated canister in liquid nitrogen for storage at -196° C. The sleeves permit easier removal of the cane and help keep ampules in place in storage, but are not essential if storage space is a problem. Frozen specimens are subsequently stored in an 'open' canister in liquid nitrogen, as for straws.

V. *Thawing of semen:* straws or ampules with frozen semen are placed in a water bath at room temperature (22° C) for thawing within five minutes. Slower thawing in air at room temperature (22° C) is also acceptable and practical. No difference has been confirmed between the two methods. Thawing in air may have an advantage with straws used as part of the insemination syringe in minimizing time and handling between thawing and insemination. Both containers are wiped dry before opening.

Straws are opened by cutting off one end with scissors, touching this end to the inside of a 0.5-dram shell vial and cutting the upper end to allow semen to run out. If straws are to be used in the special insemination syringe, the nylon plug would be in place during filling and sealing. After thawing, both ends are cut and the open straw with its plug toward the plunger end is placed in the inseminator syringe.

Ampules are opened by pressure on prescored rings and semen is transferred by a syringe or medicine dropper to a shell vial and then to an insemination device, or directly into an insemination device, as dectated by the insemination technique.

13. CONCLUDING REMARKS

Four salient factors will determine the degree to which a potentially dramatic role of cryobanking in AIH will be realized. These are:

A. The medical and lay acceptance and wider application of AIH in cases in which husband's semen is of high quality and fertile but other physical, psychological or emotional factors are responsible for his infertility;

B. The use of ever-increasing knowledge of reproductive biology both to better evaluate and define the causes of infertility and to inseminate the highest-quality semen using the best method at the optimal time in the female cycle for successful transport and fertilization;

C. The increased effectiveness of appropriate treatments of semen in vitro which are designed to improve upon semen quality by correcting, primarily, those deficiencies in characteristics of spermatozoa which are responsible for infertility;

D. The refinement of cryobiological procedures directed towards higher cryosurvival with relatively simple reproducible methods which are designed for safe and effective applications with AIH.

The key to realizing progress in cryobanking in AIH is the creation of a program concerned with continuous sharing of information for the evaluation of the four factors defined above. Physicians and investigators can accomplish this by keeping appropriate records of their clinical and research experience and, through seminars, symposia, special sessions at society meetings, questionnaires, and the like, make their findings available for exchange, evaluation and dissemination.

I trust that this brief and limited overview will not only stimulate greater use of cryobanking in AIH but will also foster greater awareness of the need for making known the results of such use, in order to realize the potentially rewarding clinical objectives of cryobanking in reproductive medicine.

REFERENCES

Alexander NJ, Kay R: Antigenicity of frozen and fresh spermatozoa. *Fertil Steril* 28:1234-1237, 1977.
Amelar RD, Hotchkiss RS: The split ejaculate: its use in the management of male infertility. *Fertil Steril* 16:46-60, 1965.
Amelar RD, Dubin L, Walsh PC: *Male infertility*, 10, Philadelphia, Saunders, 1977.
Barkay J, Zuckerman H: Further developed device for human sperm freezing by the twenty-minute method. *Fertil Steril* 29:304-308, 1978.
Barkay J, Zuckerman H, Sklan D, Gordon S: Effect of caffeine on increasing the motility of frozen human sperm. *Fertil Steril* 28:175-177, 1977.
Barwin BN: Intrauterine insemination of husband's semen. *J Reprod Fertil* 36:101-106, 1974.
Behrman SJ: Artificial insemination. In: *Progress in infertility*, Behrman SJ, Kistner RW (eds), Boston, Little, Brown, Co 1975.
Behrman SJ, Sawada Y: Heterologous and homologous inseminations with human semen frozen and stored in a liquid-nitrogen refrigerator. *Fertil Steril* 17:457-466, 1966.
Bender S: The end-results in primary sterility. *Br Med J* 2:409-413, 1952.
Black JB, Peduto JC, Servy EJ: Male factor infertility treated by isolation or progressively motile sperm: abstract. *Fertil Steril* 29:241, 1978.
Chapelle PA, Jondet M, Durand J, Grossiord A: Pregnancy of the wife of a complete paraplegic by homologous insemination after an intrathecal injection of neostigmine. *Paraplegia* 14:173-177, 1976.
Cohen MR: Intrauterine insemination. *Int J Fertil* 7:235-240, 1962.

Colton SW, Farris EJ: Low temperature preservation of human spermatozoa with practical implications. *J Urol* 80:55-56, 1958.

David G: Les banques de sperme en France. *Arch Fr Pediatr* 32:401-404, 1975.

Decker WH: Pooled and homologous (husband) semen for artificial insemination. *Infertility* 1:25-32, 1978.

Dixon RE, Buttram VC Jr, Schum CW: Artificial insemination using homologous semen: a review of 158 cases. *Fertil Steril* 27:647-654, 1976.

Dmowski WP, Gaynor L, Lawrence M, Rao R, Scommegna A: AIH with oligospermic semen separated on albumin columns. *Fertil Steril* 31:58-63, 1979.

Eckerling B: Sterility due to oligospermia and hypokinesis of the sperm: a new method of treatment. *Fertil Steril* 11:475-479, 1960.

Eliasson R, Lindholmer C: Distribution and properties of spermatozoa in different fractions of split ejaculates. *Fertil Steril* 23:252-256, 1972.

Ericsson RJ: Isolation and storage of progressively motile human sperm. *Andrologia* 9:111-114, 1977.

Fabricant JD, Boue J, Boue A: Genetic studies on spontaneous abortion. *Contemp Ob Gyn* 11:73-79, 1978.

Farris EJ, Murphy DP: The characteristics of the two parts of the partitioned ejaculate and the advantages of its use for intrauterine insemination. *Fertil Steril* 11:465-469, 1960.

Finegold WJ: *Artificial insemination*, ch 13, Springfield, Thomas, 1976.

Gasser G, Ita H, Mossig H, Schmid R, Schneider W: Experiences with AIH of native and frozen human semen. Presented at the first int symp AIH on male subfertility, Bordeaux, 1978.

Glass RH, Ericsson RJ: Intrauterine insemination of isolated motile sperm. *Fertil Steril* 29:535-538, 1978.

Glass RH, Golbus MS: Habitual abortion. *Fertil Steril* 29:257-269, 1978.

Granzow J: Biologische, serologische und pharmakologische Untersuchungen an den Spermien des Meerschweinchens und des Menschen. *Arch Gynäk* 148:149-234, 1932.

Guttmacher AF: The role of artificial insemination in the treatment of sterility. *Obstet Gynecol Survey* 15:767-785, 1960.

Hani M: The therapeutic value of artificial insemination with husband's semen. *Jap J Fertil Steril* 5:126-137, 1960.

Hanson FM, Rock J: Artificial insemination with husband's sperm. *Fertil Steril* 2:162-174, 1951.

Harrison RF: Insemination of husband's semen with or without the addition of caffeine. *Fertil Steril* 29:532-534, 1978.

Hartman CG: Correlations among criteria of semen quality. *Fertil Steril* 16:632-637, 1965.

Hirakawa W: Über den Einfluss des Prostatasekretes und der Samenflüssigkeit auf die Vitalität der Spermatozoen. *Biochem Zeitschr* 24:291-309, 1909.

Janczewski Z: Wyniki sztucznego zaptodnienia nasieniem meza w przypadkach obnizonej jego ptodnosci. *Ginekol Pol* 46:877-880, 1975, English summary.

Jecht EW, Poon Ch: Preparation of sperm free seminal plasma from human semen. *Fertil Steril* 26:1-5, 1975.

Joel CA: The role of spermatozoa in habitual abortion. *Fertil Steril* 6:459-464, 1955.

Kapetanakis E, Rao R, Dmowski WP, Scommegna A: Conception following insemination with a freeze-preserved retrograde ejaculate. *Fertil Steril* 29:360-363, 1978.

Kaskarelis D, Comminos A: A critical evaluation of homologous artificial insemination. *Int J Fertil* 4:38-41, 1959.

Keswani SG, Clitheroe HJ: Artificial insemination homologous for sub-fertility with frozen and fresh sperm concentrates. Presented at the first international symposium on AIH and male subfertility, Bordeaux, 1978.

Kihlman BA: *Caffeine and chromosomes*, Amsterdam, Elsevier, 1977.

Kleegman SJ, Kaufman SA: *Infertility in women*, Oxford, Blackwell, 1966.

Ledward RS, Crich J, Symonds EM, Cotton RE: The management of oligospermia by freezing and concentration of semen. *IRCS J Med Sci* 5:537, 1977.

MacLeod J, Gold RZ: The male factor in fertility and infertility IX: semen quality in relation to accidents of pregnancy. *Fertil Steril* 8:36-49, 1957.

Mastroianni L Jr, Laberge JL, Rock J: Appraisal of the efficacy of artificial insemination with husband's sperm and evaluation of insemination technics. *Fertil Steril* 8:260-266, 1957.

Mettenleiter M: The sperm and artificial fecundation in man and animal. *Arch Gynäk* 126:251-290, 1925.

Moghissi KS, Gruber JS, Evans S, Yanez J: Homologous artificial insemination. *Am J Obstet Gynecol* 129:909-915, 1977.

Nagase H, Niwa T: Deep freezing bull semen in concentrated pellet form. In: *Fifth international congress on animal reproduction and artificial insemination*, Trento, Italy, 1964, p 410.

Nakamura M: *Homologous AI: personal experience. Matern Infanc* 32:52-70, 1973.

Nakamura M: Artificial insemination and frozen semen. Presented at the first international symposium on AIH and male subfertility, Bordeaux, 1978.

Nakamura MS, Ramos RM: Frozen human semen: a new simplified technique of cryopreservation. In: *Recent advances in human reproduction*, Campos da Paz A, Drill VA, Hayashi M, Rodrigues W, Schally AV (eds), Amsterdam, Excerpta Medica, 1975, p 66-69.

Parez-Palaez M, Cohen MR: The split ejaculate in homologous insemination. *Int J Fertil* 10:25-30, 1965.

Parish WE, Ward A: Studies on cervical mucus and serum from infertile women. *J Obstet Gynaec Br Comm* 75:1089-1100, 1968.

Paulson JD, Polakowski KL: Isolation and storage of progressively motile human sperm. *Andrologia* 9-111-114, 1977.

Payne S, Skeels RF: Fertility as evaluated by artificial insemination. *Fertil Steril* 5:32-39, 1954.

Rosin S: The role of seminal plasma in motility of spermatozoa: therapeutic insemination with husband's semen in heterologous seminal plasma. *Acta Med Orient* 17:1-7, 1958.

Rubin A: Studies in human reproduction V: the relationship of type of seminal deficiency to difficulty of conception, based on experience in five hundred inseminations. *Fertil Steril* 12:581-585, 1961.

Rubin SO, Andersson L, Bostrom K: Deep freeze preservation of normal and pathologic human semen. *Scand J Urol Nephrol* 3:144-150, 1969.

Russell JK: Oligospermia and pregnancy: study of 34 cases. *J Obst Gynaec Brit Emp* 61:213-215, 1954.

Russell JK: Artificial insemination (husband) in the management of childlessness. *Lancet* 2:1223-1225, 1960.

Sawada Y: The preservation of human semen by deep freezing. *Int J Fertil* 9:525-532, 1964.

Schellen AMCM: *Artificial insemination in the human*, Houston, Elsevier 1957.

Schill WB: Kallikrein. In: *Kininogenases*, Haberland GL, Rohen JW, Suzuki T (eds), Stuttgart, Schattauer, 1977.

Schoenfeld CY, Amelar RD, Dubin L: Stimulation of ejaculated human spermatozoa by caffeine. *Fertil Steril* 26:158-161, 1975.

Sherman JK: Research on frozen human semen: past, present and future. *Fertil Steril* 15:485-499, 1964.

Sherman JK: Synopsis of the use of frozen human semen since 1964: state of the art of human semen banking. *Fertil Steril* 24:397-412, 1973.

Sherman JK: Clinical use of frozen human semen. *Transplant Proc 8* (Suppl 1):165-170, 1976.

Sherman JK: Cryopreservation of human semen. In: *Techniques of human andrology*, Hafez ESE (ed), Amsterdam, North-Holland Publishing, 1977.

Shields FE: Artificial insemination as related to the female. *Fertil Steril* 1:271-280, 1950.

Sillo-Seidl G: Treatment of oligospermia by freezing and concentrating semen. *Int J Fertil* 17:183-184, 1972.

Sillo-Seidl G: Different ways of homologous insemination. Presented at the first international symposium on AIH and male subfertility, Bordeaux, 1978.

Speichinger JP, Mattox JH: Homologous artificial insemination and oligospermia. *Fertil Steril* 27:135-138, 1976.

Steiman RP, Taymor ML: Artificial insemination homologous and its role in the management of infertility. *Fertil Steril* 28:146-150, 1977.

Swyer GIM: Discussion of male infertility. *Proc R Soc Med* 46:835-838, 1953.

Swyer GIM: Results of artificial insemination (husband). *J Reprod Fertil* 2:11-16, 1961.

Ulstein M: Fertility of husbands at homologous insemination. *Acta Obstet Gynecol Scand* 52:5-8, 1973.

Usherwood MM, Halim A, Evans PR: Artificial insemination (a.i.h.) for sperm antibodies and oligospermia. *Br J Urol* 48:499-503, 1976.

Warner MP: Artficial insemination: review after thirty-two years' experience. *NY State J Med* 74:2358-2361, 1974.

Weller VJ: Ergebnisse und Erfahrungen mit der artifiziellen maritogenen Insemination als Möglichkeit der Behandlung steriler Ehen. *Zentralbl Gynaekol* 98:151-157, 1976.

White RM, Glass RH: Intrauterine insemination with husband's semen. *Obstet Gynecol* 47:119-121, 1976.

Whitelaw MJ: Use of the cervical cap to increase fertility in cases of oligospermia. *Fertil Steril* 1:33-39, 1950.

15. REPEATED FREEZE-THAWING FOR ASSESSMENT OF SEMEN FREEZABILITY

A.H. ANSARI

According to our experience, as well as that of others (Behrman and Sawada 1966; Steinberger and Smith 1973) artificial insemination with frozen semen provides fewer successful pregnancies than insemination with fresh specimens. The bulk of available information (Sherman 1973; Behrman 1973) further indicates that variabilities exist in sperm freezability, some samples withstanding the stress of the freeze-thawing procedure better than others. To identify semen specimens with preserved fecundity following freeze storage, the author has utilized the recovery rate of spermatozoa motility after repeated freeze-thawing as an index of sperm freeze-preservability with impressive results.

1. TECHNIQUE

Donor semen after complete analysis was mixed with glycerol (10% by volume) and the mixture was divided into four equal portions. Specimens were then frozen over the vapor of liquid nitrogen according to the method of Sherman (1963). After freezing, each portion was placed in a properly labeled metal cane and the canes rapidly transferred into a numbered canister within the liquid-nitrogen tank. Repeated freeze-thawing (RFT) was then performed on each portion according to the following schedule: (1) immediate repeated freeze-thawing; (2) repeated freeze-thawing at monthly intervals; (3) repeated freeze-thawing at three-months intervals; and (4) repeated freeze-thawing at six-months intervals. Thawing was accomplished by leaving the sample at room temperature for a period of approximately twenty minutes. A droplet of the thawed specimen was examined for motility under high power and the motility recovery was calculated (to the nearest 5%) according to the equation:

$$\text{Motility recovery rate} = \frac{\% \text{ motile spermatozoa after thawing} \times 100}{\% \text{ motile spermatozoa prior to freezing}}$$

Samples showing a greater than 50% motility recovery rate were refrozen, stored, and reexamined after thawing at the designated time intervals. Freeze-thawing of the specimen was then repeated until loss of greater than 50% motility, i.e., a sample with pre- and post-freeze motility of 80% and 55% respectively yields a motility recovery rate of 65%, and, therefore, it is refrozen. A post-thaw motility of 33% following second freeze-thawing of this sample provides a motility recovery rate of 50% according to the equation $(33 \times 100)/65 = 50$, therefore, it is refrozen-thawed for the third time and so forth.

2. RESULTS

In general, freeze-thawings resulted in decreased sperm motility for all specimens. In addition, distinct differences were observed between various specimens. When subjected to the stress of the repeated freeze-thawing procedure, some samples preserved their motility better than others.

Table 1 demonstrates the result of RFT of 23 specimens with excellent semen analysis scores (count $>45 \times 10^6$, motility $>75\%$, viability $>75\%$ and normal morphology $>75\%$). Nearly half of the specimens lost more than 50% of their motility after second immediate freeze-thawing and only three specimens retained 50% or more motility recovery rate after the third repeated freeze-thawing (two were eliminated after the fourth and one after the sixth freeze-thawing).

A sharp decline in motility recovery following long-term frozen storage (six months) was also a common occurrence, with only two samples preserving a better than 50% motility recovery rate after a second FT of six-months interval (Table 1).

Table 1. Results of RFT of 23 specimens with excellent scores.

Freeze-thawing interval	No. of specimens retaining > 50% motility in response to RFT:			
	once	twice	three times	>three times
Immediate	19	11	5	3
Monthly	17	10	3	1
Three months	16	6	1	0
six months	10	2	0	0

Artificial inseminations with frozen semen of these 23 donors resulted in 11 pregnancies. One pregnancy was achieved from a donor whose specimen showed less than 50% motility recovery rate after first freeze-thawing. The remaining 10 pregnancies resulted from 6 donors (one donor achieving 3 pregnancies, two donors each producing two pregnancies, and the other 3 pregnancies resulting from 3 different donors) with satisfactory motility recovery according to immediate RFT. It is interesting to note that the semen from donors producing three and two pregnancies retained greater than 50% motility recovery after three freeze-thawing procedures.

It should be mentioned that samples with poor motility recovery rate following immediate freeze-thawing also showed less than 50% recovery rate after monthly, three-months and six-months freeze-thawing intervals. In addition, significant reduction in motility recovery was encountered after prolonged frozen storage (six months), nearly half of the samples losing greater than 50% motility recovery rate in the first freeze-thawing process. It is noteworthy that the majority of the samples with satisfactory motility recovery rate following immediate repeated freeze-thawing also showed the ability to withstand the stress of prolonged cryopreservation. In contrast to samples with excellent scores, the specimens with a fair-to-good score (count 20-40 $\times$ 10^6, motility 60-70%, viability 60-70%, normal morphology 60-70%) withstood the stress of repeated freeze-thawing procedures poorly, especially after prolonged storage (Table 2). Three pregnancies were achieved from the frozen semen of three donors in this group of cases with all three donors having good semen analysis scores and a motility recovery rate of greater than 50% after the second immediate freeze-thawing.

Table 2. Results of RFT of 15 specimens with fair-good scores.

Freeze-thawing interval	No. of specimens retaining 50% motility in response to RFT:			
	once	twice	three times	>three times
immediate	7	3	1	1
Monthly	6	2	1	0
Three months	6	1	1	0
Six months	4	1	0	0

Table 3 illustrates the results of repeated freeze-thawings of oligospermic specimens. The results clearly demonstrate poor frozen storage of these specimens. Two pregnancies ensued following months of homologous inseminations with concentrated frozen semen of two oligospermic males with good semen quality in this group of cases. Admittedly, the possibility of naturally occurring conception cannot be ruled out with certainty since couples maintained normal sexual relationship during the entire course of artificial insemination.

If confirmed by additional studies this observation may advantageously provide an effective method of selecting suitable donors for prolonged frozen storage.

Table 3. Pregnancy outcome of oligospermic specimens according to 50% motility recovery following immediate RFT.

Type of specimen	No. of specimens	Post-RFT motility recovery		Pregnancy outcome*
		1-3	>3	
Oligospermic Specimens with fair-good score	14	4	0	2
Oligospermic specimens with poor score**	17	0	0	0

  * AIH with concentrated frozen semen
** Count: $<20 \times 10^6$; motility: $<60\%$; viability: $<60\%$; normal morphology: $<60\%$.

3. DISCUSSION

Despite successful frozen storage of human semen and its practical advantages for artificial insemination (Table 4), the future fertilizing capacity of such a sample is never guaranteed. Furthermore, semen specimens of normal quality not uncommonly fail to reproduce following cryopreservation.

The process of freeze-thawing undoubtedly results in physical and/or chemical alterations in the spermatozoa (Ackerman 1968; Friberg and Nilsson 1971; Pederson and Lebech 1971; Sherman 1967), the degree of which not only varies from species to species (Mixner and Wiggin 1964, Cassou 1972; Salamon and Visser 1974), as shown in superior results in cattle freeze-preservation in sharp contrast to poor results in swine and sheep, but also among the specimens of the same species, including man (Sherman 1963; Behrman 1973). According to the results of repeated freeze-thawing recorded here, the magnitude of the adverse effect of freeze-preservation appears to be in direct relationship to the quality of the specimens. As mentioned before, the samples of inferior quality withstood the stress of repeated freeze-thawing procedures very poorly, producing a very limited number of pregnancies. The post-thaw motility recovery rate of cryo-preserved semen had also according to Ulstein (1973), a direct correlation with the pre-freeze condition of the sample. Ulstein's studies showed significant reduction in sperm motility and penetrability within the cervical mucus of cryopreserved semens of poor quality. Similarly, Behrman states that when the post-thaw motility recovery exceeds 60% of the original motility, a 70% preg-

Table 4. Advantages of artificial insemination with frozen semen.

1. Readily available
2. Wider selection of specimens
3. Avoidance of inconvenience and unnecessary expense
4. Large-volume insemination practical
5. May provide avenues for management of male infertility

nancy rate may be expected, in contrast to a 30% successful conception when the sample exhibits less than 60% motility recovery (Behrman 1973). Obviously, other factors beside motility, such as metabolic and ultrastructural alterations, are equally important in the fertilizing capacity of the frozen-stored semen. Although post-thaw motility is usually influenced by these changes the semen may nonetheless preserve its motility despite the encountered cellular and metabolic alterations during freeze-thawing procedures.

Concurrently, according to our observations, some semen specimens fail to reproduce despite adequate motility recovery following cryopreservation. Conceivably, frozen storage may result in certain metabolic and ultrastructural changes incompatible with fertilization, without significant deleterious effect on sperm motility. However, using motility recovery rate following repeated cryopreservation as an index of fertilizing capacity, we were able to identify semen samples which yielded higher pregnancy rates.

4. SUMMARY

Despite availability of successful techniques for frozen storage of human semen, future fecundity of such a specimen is never guaranteed, and not uncommonly, a normal semen fails to result in pregnancy after frozen storage. Variability also exists among the semen samples, some specimens tolerating the stress of the semen banking process better than others.

Identification of a semen specimen with preserved fertility not only has its advantages in the field of artificial insemination, but may also have its impact in the field of family planning. Vasectomy may be readily accepted by those whose semen specimen maintains fertilizing ability following freeze-preservation. Using the repeated freeze-thawing technique as described in this report may facilitate identification of those cases in whom future fecundity may be preserved through cryopreservation of semen prior to vasectomy. Additionally, results of RFT indicate that samples with loss of motility after the second or third freezing procedure withstood poorly a long frozen storage and also provided a poor pregnancy rate.

Lastly, other factors listed in Table 5 may also influence semen freezability and post frozen-storage fecundity unfavorably.

Table 5. Factors unfavorably influencing semen freezability and post-frozen-storage fecundity.

---

1. Inferior semen analysis score
2. Unsatisfactory motility recovery following RFT
3. Prolonged duration of frozen storage
4. Oligospermic specimen
5. Prolonged interval (< 60 minutes) between collection of specimen and freezing

---

REFERENCES

Ackerman DR: The effect of cooling and freezing on the aerobic and anaerobic lactic acid production of human semen. *Fertil Steril* 19-123, 1968.
Behrman SJ, Sawada Y: Heterologous and homologous insemination with human semen frozen and stored in a liquid-nitrogen refrigerator. *Fertil Steril* 17:457, 1966.
Behrman SJ: The preservation of semen; editorial. *Fertil Steril* 24:396, 1973.
Cassou R: Development of fertility rate in terms of age of semen. *Int Congr Animal Reprod AI* 7:1421, 1972.
Friberg J, Nilsson O: Motility and morphology of human sperm after freezing in liquid nitrogen. In: *Current problem in fertility*, Ingelman Sundberg A Lunell NO (eds), New York, Plenum 1971, p 17.
Mixner JP, Wiggin SH: The effect of aging on the motility and fertility of frozen bull semen. *Int Congr Animal Reprod AI* 5:264, 1964.
Pederson H Lebech PE: Ultrastructural changes in the human spermatozoa after freezing for artificial insemination. *Fertil Steril* 22:125, 1971.
Salamon S, Visser: Fertility of ram spermatozoa frozen stored for 5 years. *J Reprod Fertil* 37:433, 1974.
Sawada Y, Ackerman DR Behrman SJ: Motility and respiration of human spermatozoa after cooling to various low temperatures. *Fertil Steril* 18:775, 1967.
Sherman JK: Improved methods of preservation of human spermatozoa by freezing and freeze-drying. *Fertil Steril* 14:49, 1963.
Sherman JK: Freeze-thaw induced latent injury as a phenomenon in cryobiology. *Cryobiology* 3:407, 1967.
Sherman JK: Synopsis of the use of frozen human semen since 1964: state of the art of human semen banking. *Fertil Steril* 24:397, 1973.
Steinberger E, Smith KD: Artificial insemination with fresh and frozen semen. *JAMA* 223:778, 1973.
Ulstein M: Fertility, motility and penetration in cervical mucus of freeze-preserved human spermatozoa. *Acta Obstet Gynecol Scand* 52:205, 1973.

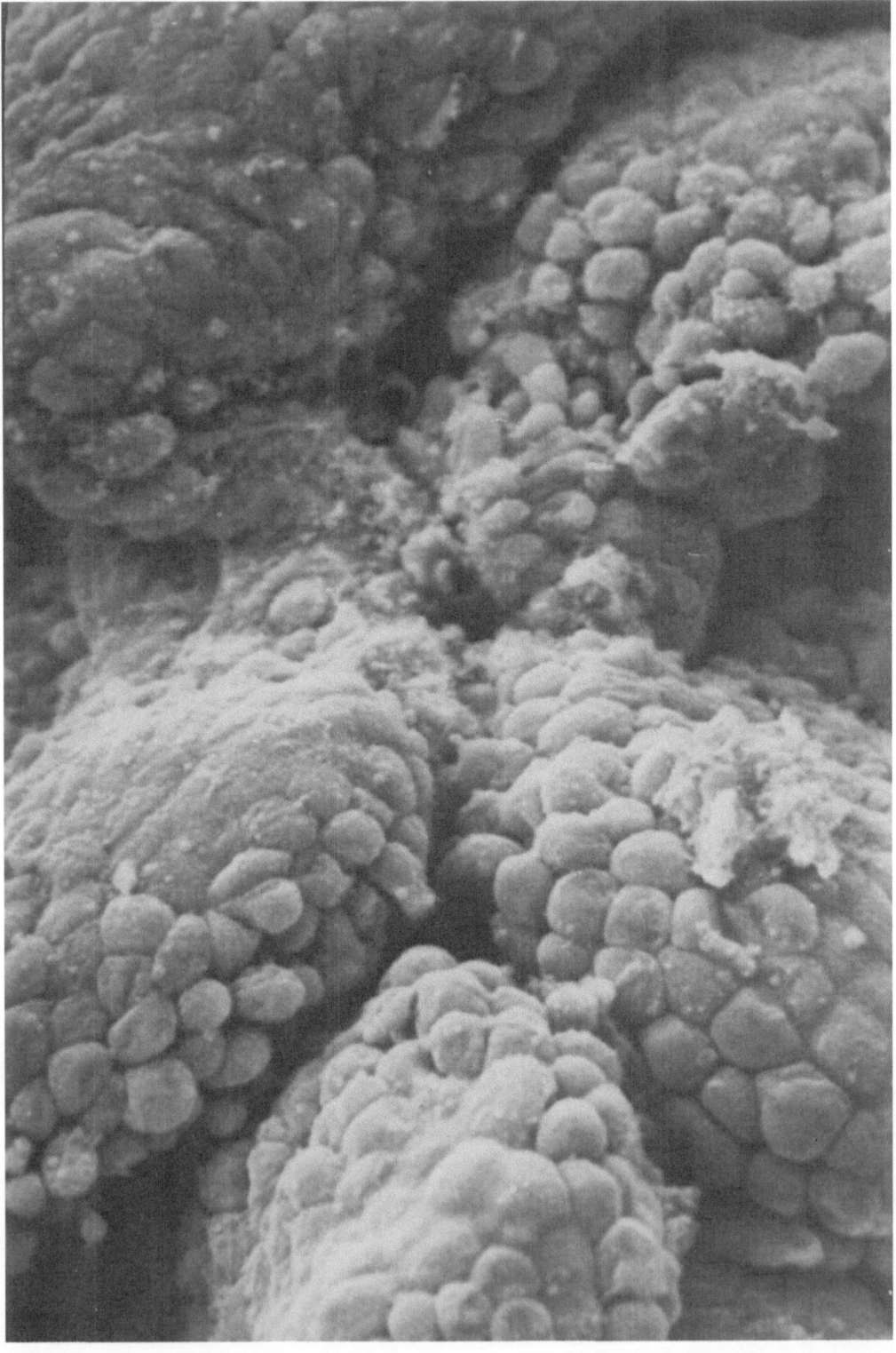

III. CLINICAL PARAMETERS OF INSEMINATION

16. INSEMINATION TECHNIQUES

J. Belaisch, J. Kremer, O. Steeno and J. Paulson

In past years, artificial insemination utilizing the husband's semen (AIH) was considered to result in almost universal failure. Recent work, however, has disclosed that this past pessimism can be replaced with a guarded and reasonable basis for optimism in certain circumstances.

AIH (artificial insemination homologous) is a psychologically safe procedure, but one with limited application. Less than 10% of infertile couples associated with a male factor leading to infertility should be considered for this procedure (Beck 1977). Insemination of a normospermic specimen with normal semen parameters into a physiologically normal female having a normal postcoital test is not usually indicated.

The most frequently performed technique in artificial insemination is intra-cervical insemination. As this procedure implies, semen is deposited in the cervical canal and there is almost always a partial backflow into the vaginal vault. This method is useful in many cases; however, other techniques may yield higher pregnancy rates in certain instances for specific indications. Besides intracervical insemination, intrauterine, vaginal and cervical-cap techniques offer true therapeutic possibilities.

1. INDICATIONS

The largest number of patients undergoing AIH do so because of oligospermia and/or diminished motility (Table 1). Problems with the delivery of the semen also constitute a large percentage of the inseminations that are performed. Impotence and premature ejaculation are two of the major psychological problems for which AIH can yield good pregnancy rates. Causes of infertility due to anatomic abnormalities (such as vaginal anomalies, retrograde ejaculation and hypospadias) which prevent deposition of the semen in the vagina to allow penetration through the cervical mucus are also successfully treated by artificial insemination.

Ejaculates with low semen volumes but with otherwise normal parameters including motility, sperm density and morphology may be associated with reduced fertility because of dilution of the semen and loss of protection against

Table 1. Indications for artificial insemination homologous (AIH).

Male	Female
Oligo-asthenospermia	Vaginismus
Low Semen volume	Thick, impermeable cervical mucus
Retrograde ejaculation	Cervical stenosis
Impotence	Normal-appearing but hostile cervical mucus
Hypospadias	
Irradiation of testes for tumor	Retroflexion of uterus
(previous cryopreservation)	
Premature ejaculation	

vaginal acidity. If several negative postcoital tests are obtained, artificial insemination may prove fruitful. Poor postcoital tests with an otherwise normal assessment can often be overcome by special insemination procedures.

2. METHODS OF INSEMINATION

There are four major methods of insemination now employed: intrauterine, intracervical (cervical), vaginal, and cervical cap (Figure 1). Often two of the methods, such as intracervical and vaginal, are used simultaneously. The actual insemination is the culmination of the procedure that has involved male and female evaluations, establishing an ovulatory pattern and inseminating on the proper days.

2.1. Intrauterine insemination

It is difficult to determine spermatozoal survival in the different compartments of the human female genital tract because investigations seldom provide reliable results. The difficulty is that the presence of motile spermatozoa in a certain compartment does not mean that the spermatozoa have always been there since coitus or insemination took place. When motile spermatozoa are detected in the uterine cavity 24 hours after coitus (Belonoschkin 1949) these spermatozoa may have arrived there from the cervix just five minutes earlier. Motile spermatozoa recovered from the oviduct 60-80 hours after intercourse (Ahlgren 1969) may have left the uterine cavity only seconds earlier. Motile spermatozoa collected from the pouch of Douglas (Horne and Thibault 1962) were possibly still in the oviduct when the preparations for the cul-de-sac puncture were made. There are still many unanswered questions regarding sperm survival in the human female genital tract. It is generally assumed, however, that the vagina is the area of the female with the greatest hostility towards spermatozoa, and that the cervical

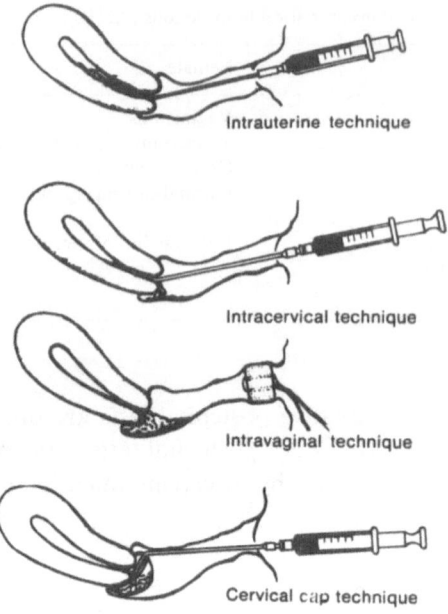

Figure 1. Methods of artificial insemination.

crypts, when filled with normal preovulatory cervical mucus, are the most favorable environments for them.

Although the presence of phagocytes supports the supposition that the uterine cavity is a hostile compartment, some investigators believe that the endometrial glands may serve as a secondary storage site for spermatozoa (Moghissi 1977). The area of the utero-tubal junction, in particular, should act as a sperm reservoir (Hafez and Black 1969). Even though it would seem logical that the milieu in the Fallopian tube should be favorable to the spermatozoa, there are indications that the degree of hospitality is much less than in the cervical crypts (Hafez 1976).

The passage from the uterine cavity into the tubes occurs rapidly (Fordney Settlage et al. 1973), thereby relegating the time the spermatozoa remain in the uterus to a short one, so the milieu is much less important than for a stay of longer duration. Because of these facts and suppositions, intrauterine insemination appears to be an unphysiological procedure. There are also a number of disadvantages in comparison with the other techniques. Introduction of the cannula may prove difficult and the process may be associated with bleeding and uterine cramps. Placing foreign objects into the cavity can possibly cause pelvic infections. Because it is felt that the cervical crypts act as a reservoir for spermatozoa, allowing release of a small but continuous number, it is possible that by directly placing spermatozoa into the uterus, there is a lack of protection for long periods of time as can be afforded by the cervical mucus. Because the passage of the spermatozoa from the uterine cavity into the oviducts occurs rapidly, the chance of fertilization decreases if the woman has not ovulated.

Nevertheless, some authors have reported reasonable success with few or no complications with intrauterine insemination (Farris and Murphy 1960; Cohen 1962; Barwin 1974; White and Glass 1976).

In order to minimize trauma and offer a painless introduction of the cannula, the instrument should have the following properties:

1. It should have a rounded, smooth tip.
2. The tip should be thin enough to pass through the internal os.
3. The first 2 cm of the cannula must be flexible enough to follow the curvature of the uterine wall during introduction into the uterine cavity.
4. The second part of the cannula must be rigid in order to overcome slight resistance.
5. The length of the cannula should not exceed 5 cm and the opening should be located on the side of the instrument.

The 5-cm end piece of a ch 6-8 rubber catheter, splinted over a distance of 4 cm with a rigid polyethylene cannula fulfills these requirements. If the cervix and the uterine cavity are of normal length, the tip of the catheter does not reach the utero-tubal junction (Figure 2a).

If the uterus is small and the distance from the external cervical os to the utero-tubal junction is less than 5 cm, the lateral opening of the catheter prevents direct intratubal insemination (Figure 2b). The tip of the catheter blocks the entrance of the tube and the semen spreads in the cleft between the anterior and the posterior wall of the uterine cavity and does not enter the tubes. If no more than 0.2 ml of semen is introduced, the chance of indirect intratubal insemination, due to myometrial contractions, is small.

In order to prevent infection, fresh semen is collected in such a way that contamination with micro-organisms is minimized. The patients are asked to collect the semen by masturbation and to wash their hands and penis prior to this. Even with these precautions, bacterial contamination can and does occur (Wu 1957; Kremer 1978).

Micturition just before ejaculation must be avoided to prevent the addition of urine to the semen. In order to prevent uterine cramps, the first part of a split ejaculate is used if feasible. This contains a much lower concentration of prostaglandins than the second part, another advantage of utilizing split ejaculates is that semen quality, in terms of sperm density and motility, is, in general, better than in the second part of an ejaculate.

The safety of this system was demonstrated in 30 women scheduled for hysterosalpingography, in whom the introduction of 2 ml of lipidol in the uterine cavity by means of the splinted rubber catheter did not result in any filling of the

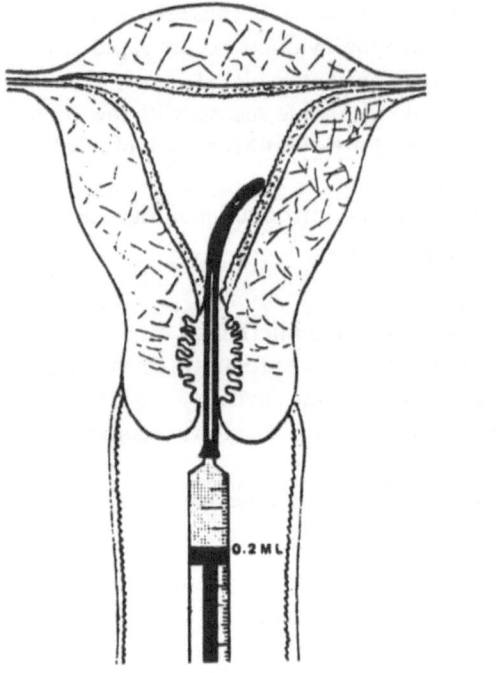

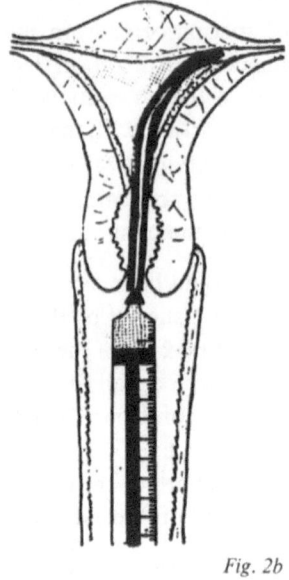

Fig. 2b

Fig. 2a

Fig. 2a. Tuberculine syringe, filled with 0.2 ml of the first part of a split ejaculate and provided with the 5 cm long end piece of a paediatric rubber catheter (charriere 6-8).The catheter is splinted with a rigid polyethylene canula (diameter 1.34 mm).

Fig. 2b. If the uterine cavity is small and the distance from the external cervical os to the uterotubal junction is less than 5 cm, the lateral opening of the catheter prevents direct intratubal insemination.

tubes. When the tip of the catheter entered a tubal corner of the uterus, the tube remained empty after introduction of 0.2 ml of the contrast medium (Kremer 1978).

Checking for the possibility of spermatozoal antibody formation has only recently been done (Kremer 1978), even though intrauterine inseminations have been performed for many years. Table 2 demonstrates that in the majority of patients there was little or no increase in titres. In only 13% was there an increase in the titres, and these patients also had a strongly positive SCMC test (Kremer and Jager 1976) in addition to the sperm agglutinating activity of the blood serum.

This method of insemination is performed by inserting the cannula through the internal os into the uterine cavity after grasping the anterior lip of the cervix with a tenaculum. Through this cannula 0.2-0.3 cc of either whole semen, split ejaculate of buffered spermatozoal solution is injected slowly. This procedure is performed only for limited indications.

Table 2. Effect of intrauterine inseminations on sperm agglutinin titre in serum of 33 infertile women, all but one of whom were inseminated once or twice during six cycles.

Number of women	SCMC test	TAT titre of serum	
		before insemination	after insemination
24	neg	≤4	≤4
5	neg	4-8	4-16
1	+++	16	256
1	+++	16	128
1*	+++	64	≥512
1	+++	128	1024

* pregnant during first insemination cycle; second TAT titre measured during first trimester of pregnancy (Kremer 1978).

2.2. Intracervical insemination

In cases where there is cervical stenosis or cervical mucus impermeable to sperm a cannula can be inserted midway between the external os and the internal os and as the semen is slowly instilled, the cannula is slowly withdrawn. The excess semen runs out of the canal and falls into the vaginal vault.

2.3. Vaginal insemination

This involves depositing the semen in the vagina. The patient is placed in 10 to 15 degrees of Trendelenburg. The cervical os may or may not be placed in contact with the semen. If it is, the speculum can be adjusted so that the cervix is dipped into the semen pool in the vagina. Occasionally a small amount of semen is placed in the os and the remainder is put into the vaginal vault. The patient remains in the Trendelenburg position for twenty minutes. This method should be utilized in homologous insemination only for problems of delivery of the semen.

2.4. Cervical-cap insemination

This technique is a modification of the cervical and the vaginal insemination methods. The cervical cap is a plastic cup into which the whole semen or split ejaculate is placed. This method seems to imitate the natural process most closely while eliminating the hostile vaginal environment.

Two designs for cervical-cap insemination are now used. The first is a plastic cap with no stem into which the semen or split ejaculate is placed prior to the cap being put on the cervix. By removing the upper blade of the speculum, the cap is slid down on the lower blade and when the cervix is encountered, the cap is pushed into place on the cervix and remains there because a slight vacuum is created and the vaginal wall helps to hold it secure. The cap with a stem is brought close to the cervix and, with the use of a small pump under constant negative pressure, the cap is applied to the cervix. The vacuum is maintained through a clip and 1-3 ml of semen is injected into the catheter, followed by 1.5 ml air. The air helps to empty the tubal content as well as allow easier release of the cap.

The cervical cap may be removed anywhere from 4 h after insemination to the next morning. For caps without stems, removal is performed by dislodging the cap from the cervix with a finger and pulling the cap out of the vagina. If the cap has a stem, the rolling clip is undone, thereby releasing the vacuum and the cap can then be removed from the vagina.

An advantage of the cervical-cap method over the intracervical method is that during the latter, foreign material is being introduced in the cervix while the cervical cap allows for the normal mechanism of penetration and infiltration of spermatozoa and it prevents leucocytes from infiltration into the endocervix after application. This is important if one has to inseminate repeatedly during the same cycle.

2.5. Intraconjugal inseminations (auto-insemination)

Because the strict chronological requirements for artificial insemination present hindrances to the social and psychological lives of couples involved as well as a financial burden, an alternative to the procedure being performed in the sterile atmosphere of the doctor's office can be accomplished. Intraconjugal insemination, or auto-insemination, is the insemination of the husband's semen into the cervix or the vagina of the wife by the husband himself in the privacy of their home. There is no doubt that this procedure dehumanizes the act of love and reaps potential psychological problems. However, for mature couples who understand and can cope with this, this procedure may have potential reward. There are four theoretical areas in which it could be used: (1) vaginismus of the wife, (2) sexual difficulties of the husband, (3) anatomic malformations of the husband, and (4) deficient production of spermatozoa due to various causes. The first two indications represent psychological problems which must be handled jointly with the opinion and advice of a qualified psychotherapist. In these cases, and for problems of anatomic malformation, the semen is deposited from a syringe into the fornix of the vagina for two to three consecutive days before a temperature rise is seen. If a sample is oligo-astheno-teratospermic, insemination intracervically or with a cervical cap would offer better results (perhaps with a split ejaculate).

Husbands can be taught to use a speculum and learn to recognize the cervical os. Using the basal body temperature chart, and by recognizing the change of the cervix and the preovulatory mucus change, the husband can inseminate at the appropriate times with his own sperm. The husbands can then be instructed in placing a cervical cap with semen on the cervix or introducing a cannula (a Braun cannula has been recommended) just inside the external os (1/2 cm) and inject approximately 0.1 ml every 2 or 3 minutes allowing the highly motile spermatozoa to make their way up into the mucus. The process should be repeated every day or every other day until ovulation time has passed. The couple must, also, be instructed not to inseminate until after liquefaction has occurred. A post-insemination test can be performed the day following the first insemination by having the physician do a Sims-Hühner test to note the presence or absence of motile spermatozoa. This is also a check on whether the insemination was accomplished satisfactorily.

3. TIMING

An average day of ovulation can be calculated from the basal body temperature charts of the three previous menstrual cycles. If the mean day of ovulation is several days different on any of the single months, it may be necessary to regulate ovulation. Unlike AID (donor insemination), where inseminating two or three times per cycle around ovulation time is satisfactory, AIH for non-psychological problems is a process that involves semen of questioned quality. However, since the couple does not have to pay for donor semen, multiple inseminations can be performed to help offset the quality of the semen. Insemination can begin two days before the conjectured ovulation. If intrauterine insemination is done, the procedure can be repeated frequently until ovulation occurs (because of the suspected shortened fertile period inside the uterine cavity). For other procedures insemination should be performed every two days until a rise in temperature has taken place. The day after the first insemination a Sims-Hühner (post-coital) test is done; AIH should be continued only if a sufficient number of motile spermatozoa are found in the cervical mucus after 24 hours.

4. CLINICAL SUCCESS

Success with homologous insemination is dependent on the primary cause of infertility. If the semen is of good quantity and quality, such as in inseminations for psychological disorders, anatomic problems or low volume, then AIH has good success. If the semen has oligospermia and decreased mobility, the results of AIH are poor. It is necessary to have inseminations during an adequate time interval of at least six months with several inseminations each cycle before abandoning this procedure. The addition of pharmacological agents to the ejaculate, filtration of the semen by glass wool and serum albumin columns, and other in vitro treatments of semen including the use of split ejaculates prior to insemination are discussed in great depth in another chapter.

Retrograde ejaculation has been approached in several successful ways. Premasturbated catheterization is followed by washing the bladder with a nutrient fluid allowing several ml to remain in the bladder. This is then followed by masturbation and a second catheterization to obtain a specimen. This was the most common way spermatozoa were recovered in the past in order to inseminate (Hotchkiss et al. 1955). Alkalinizing with oral bicarbonate, obtaining a postcoital urine and centrifuging in order to obtain a sample to inseminate seems to have less of an adverse psychological effect and less stress than a technique involving catherization, and successful results are seen (Glezerman et al. 1976). The semen can even be recovered from retrograde ejaculators, cryopreserved and used for insemination at a later time with successful pregnancies resulting (Kapetanakis et al. 1978).

Results from intraconjugal inseminations have been surprisingly satisfying. Although only a small series of 55 patients has been reported, 20% achieved pregnancy without any psycho-sexual problems (Belaisch 1978). Ten of the eleven delivered normal-term children. The eleventh ended in a stillborn with trisomy 23 (mother was 38).

Intrauterine inseminations have been used successfully when cervical mucus, not amenable to therapy, is too viscid for sperm penetration and when sperm are immobilized in normal mucus. Two authors have pregnancy rates of 55% for these indications (Barwin 1974; White and Glass 1976). Poor results are obtained if insemination is performed using subfertile semen specimens or for couples who have both poor postcoital tests and poor in vitro cervical mucus penetration tests; however, results obtained in couples with normal semen and a good penetration test, but a poor postcoital test, and results with couples with unexplained infertility, are good, with a 55% pregnancy rate (Kremer 1978).

This indicates that a normal interaction between spermatozoa and cervical mucus is favorable for conception after intrauterine insemination. This might suggest that after intrauterine insemination a number of spermatozoa return to the mucus in the cervical crypts. If they find a favorable milieu there, they have a much better chance for a long sperm life than their comrades in the uterine cavity, in the oviducts, and in the peritoneal cavity. If this is true, the success of intrauterine insemination is, in a number of cases, due to indirect intracervical insemination via the internal cervical os. But what is then the advantage of intrauterine insemination over intracervical insemination? Is it possibly a better sperm colonization of the cervical crypts in the neighbourhood of the internal os? Whatever it may be, in couples where the interaction between spermatozoa and cervical mucus is thoroughly disturbed, intrauterine insemination is the only possible method with a chance of success.

Because the milieu in the uterine cavity is supposed to be relatively hostile to spermatozoa and the stay in the oviducts is short, one must try to perform the intrauterine insemination in these couples a short time before ovulation. Because this is difficult, the success rate of intrauterine inseminations in couples where the cervical mucus cannot offer a safe shelter to spermatozoa is rather disappointing.

Artificial inseminations by the cervical-cap technique and/or intracervical inseminations have been previously reported. In one series using split ejaculates, a pregnancy rate of 46% was achieved for couples who underwent six or more cycles of insemination, but a disappointing spontaneous abortion rate of 50% was observed (Moghissi et al. 1977). A different series reported a pregnancy rate of 20.8% (Nunley et al. 1978); however, if the females are divided into normally fertile and those with infertility factors, the group of women with normal fertility had a higher pregnancy rate (50%) than those with other problems (13.9%). The spontaneous abortion rate in this group of patients was 35.7%. Others have shown pregnancy rates after AIH to be statistically similar between women undergoing insemination who had normal fertility – 8/29 – and women who had additional factors which could account for the infertility – 9/28 (Steiman and Taymor 1977).

A large series of 158 couples revealed a pregnancy rate of 9.5%, 15 pregnancies (Dixon et al. 1976). However, after three months, approximately half of the couples had discontinued inseminations and 113 of the 158 had dropped out by the end of the fifth cycle.

In another series of 128 women, split ejaculates and different other methods to increase sperm concentration and motility have been utilized to practice AIH. The pregnancy rate was thirty one per cent and the success rate per cycle five per cent (David et al. 1978).

Most inseminations are performed because of abnormalities in density, morphology and/or motility. Because of the increased abnormal morphology, pregnancy conception rate is low and this may explain the high abortion rate.

A different approach to AIH involves using frozen semen (Speck, personal communication, 1978), although it is well appreciated that cryopreservation decreases the motility of the sample and is usually devastating to an oligo-asthenospermic specimen. The use of a split ejaculate would help achieve a more motile specimen. By collecting and freezing the husband's semen every four to five days, and just prior to ovulation time inseminating every morning and having the couple have intercourse at night, it was felt that pregnancy rates in couples whose husbands were the predominant cause of infertility would increase. Preliminary results have demonstrated a pregnancy rate of 34% with a spontaneous abortion rate of 9%.

In a recently concluded study (Steeno 1978), 143 patients were diagnosed with an andrological indication for homologous insemination (AIH). Several patients became pregnant two or three times. The success rate in the total group treated by cervical-cap technique was 27.3%. In the group of oligozoospermia with normal motility and morphology, where split-ejaculate technique was applied, the success rate was 43.7%. In the total group of patients with an andrological indication for AIH there were 36 female patients with diminished fertility chances. From this group of 36, five became pregnant (13.9%). Omitting these 36 couples with diminished fertility chances in both partners the success rate increases from 27.3 to 32%. Four patients who had first become pregnant through artificial insemination then became pregnant spontaneously, whereas 13 patients became pregnant spontaneously after artificial insemination had failed.

Table 3 shows the number of successful inseminations with semen of diminished quality in reference to the state of semen quality of deficiency, using the

Table 3. AI with semen of diminished quality by means of the cervical-cap technique (Steeno 1978).

State of semen quality or deficiency	Split ejaculate		whole semen	
	patients treated	pregnancies obtained	patients treated	pregnancies obtained
1. Oligozoospermia	8	5	9	1
2. Asthenozoospermia	1	0	17	1
3. Oligo-asthenozoospermia	5	1	22	12
4. Oligo-teratozoospermia	1	1	6	4
5. Oligo-astheno-teratozoospermia	8	3	46	12
Total	23	10	100	30

whole ejaculate or the first part of a split ejaculate.

The most influential factor upon the success rate is the motility of the spermatozoa. Thirty percent progressive motility is thought to be necessary for reasonable conception rates.

5. CONCLUDING REMARKS

Homologous insemination is a procedure which may have good results if the patient population is carefully screened. Psychological hindrances to fertility can often be circumvented by use of this technique. In certain instances of cervical mucus hostility and even in a few cases of infertility of long duration, intrauterine inseminations have been shown to achieve surprisingly good conception rates; the exact mechanism of sperm storage or release has not yet been elucidated. For individuals with oligo-asthenospermia with a motility of at least 30%, intracervical or cervical-cap insemination techniques have been shown in some instances to allow limited conception in the female partner. Vaginal and intrauterine insemination are not warranted for these individuals.

This type of procedure is being used more and more as recognition of andrological problems becomes more prevalent. Although medical therapy and treatment of the ejaculate in vitro prior to insemination are steadily increasing, these modes of therapy are still in early stages of development and, unfortunately, do not offer spectacular results.

REFERENCES

Ahlgren M: *Migration of spermatozoa to the Fallopian tubes and the abdominal cavity in women including some immunological aspects*, Lund, Student Literatur, 1969.

Barwin BN: Intrauterine insemination of husband's semen. *J Reprod Fertil* 36:101, 1974.

Beck WW: Artificial insemination. In: *Techniques of human andrology* Hafez ESE (ed), Amsterdam, North-Holland Publishing 1977, p 421.

Belaisch J: Insémination intra-conjugale par le mari. Presented at the first international symposium on AIH and male subfertility, Bordeaux, 1978.

Belonoschkin G: *Erzeugung beim Menschen in Lichte der Spermatozoenlehre*. Stockholm, Sjobergs, 1949.

Cohen MR: Intrauterine insemination. *Int J Fertil* 7-235, 1962.

David G, Gernigon C, Kunstmann JM: Insémination artificielle avec sperme du conjoint. *J Gyn Obst Biol Repr* 7:686, 1978.

Dixon RE, Buttram VC, Schum C: Artificial insemination using homologous semen: a review of 158 cases. *Fertil Steril* 27:647, 1976.

Farris EJ, Murphy DP: The characteristics of the two parts of the partitioned ejaculate and the advantages of its use for intrauterine insemination. *Fertil Steril* 11:465, 1960.

Fordney Settlage DS, Motoshima M, Tredway DR: Sperm transport from the external cervical os to the Fallopian tubes in women: a time and quantitation study. *Fertil Steril* 24:655, 1973.

Glezerman M, Lunenfeld B, Potashnik G, Oelsner G, Beer R: Retrograde ejaculation: pathophysiologic aspects and report of two successfully treated cases. *Fertil Steril* 27:796, 1976.

Hafez ESE: Transport and survival of spermatozoa in the female reproductive tract. In: *Human semen and fertility regulation in men*, Hafez ESE (ed), St. Louis, Mosby, 1976.

Hafez ESE, Black DL: The mammalian uterotubal junction. In: *The mammalian oviduct: comparative biology and methodology*. Hafez ESE, Blandau J (eds), Chicago, University of Chicago Press, 1969.

Horne HW, Thibault J: Sperm migration through the human female reproductive tract. *Fertil Steril* 13:135, 1962.

Hotchkiss RS, Pinto AB, Kleegman S: Artificial insemination with semen recovered from the bladder. *Fertil Steril* 6:37, 1955.

Kapetanakis E, Rao R, Dmowski WP, Scommegna A: Conception following insemination with a freeze-preserved retrograde ejaculate. *Fertil Steril* 29:360, 1978.

Kremer J: A new technique for intrauterine insemination. Presented at the first international symposium on AIH and male subfertility, Bordeaux, 1978.

Kremer J, Jager S: The sperm-cervical mucus contact test: a preliminary report. *Fertil Steril* 27:335, 1976.

Moghissi KS: Sperm migration through the human cervix. In: *The uterine cervix in reproduction*, Stuttgart, Georg Thieme, 1977.

Moghissi KS, Gruber JS, Evans S, Yanez J: Homologous artificial insemination: a reappraisal. *Am J Obstet Gynecol* 129:909, 1977.

Nunley WC, Kitchin JD, Thiagarajah S: Homologous insemination. *Fertil Steril* 30:510, 1978.

Steeno O: Cervical cap technique of insemination. Presented at the first international symposium on AIH and male subfertility, Bordeaux 1978.

Steiman RP, Taymor ML: Artificial insemination homologous and its role in the management of infertility. *Fertil Steril* 28:146, 1977.

White RM, Glass RH: Intrauterine insemination with husband's semen. *Obstet Gynecol* 47:119, 1976.

Wu DH: Bacteriological studies on the semen. and experimental studies on the influences of antibiotics, crystalline penicillin potassium, dihydrostreptomycin sulfate and terramycin hydrochloride upon the semen. *Kei-O Med J* 34:509, 1957.

17. DONOR INSEMINATION VERSUS AIH

J. PAULSON and A.H. ANSARI

In recent years liberalization of abortion and effective methods of contraception have inevitably resulted in the diminishing availability of adoptable children. As a result many hopelessly infertile couples, who in the past preferred adoption to artificial insemination, have now revised their attitudes, requesting and, on occasion, even demanding artificial insemination. Presently, artificial insemination is a fully established and accepted medical procedure, performed with increasing frequency.

The possibility of impregnation by means other than natural intercourse has long been appreciated. The commentary on the Bible by Jewish scholars, the Talmud, begun shortly after the beginning of the Christian era, recognizes in several different circumstances that this could happen. The first reported use of artificial insemination in modern times was reported by Hunter after success involving a male with hypospadias in the late 1700s (Rohleder 1934; Shields 1950). In 1833 a Frenchman, Girault, is credited with the next documented report of successful inseminations. In the mid-1800s Sims published his procedure for intracervical artificial insemination in women who had poor postcoital tests. Up till this time, artificial insemination had been limited to the use of the husband's semen, but in 1890 Robert Dickinson began utilizing artificial insemination by donor semen. These inseminations were performed in great secrecy due to the non-acceptance of this procedure in the United States. Since these earliest reports, the use of artificial insemination has increased in more recent times as the interest in infertility and reproduction has grown and the availability of adoptable babies has decreased.

There are two types of artificial insemination: homologous, which uses the husband's semen, and heterologous, which utilizes semen from a donor. Homologous insemination poses no legal problems because the resulting child is the biological offspring of both husband and wife. Heterologous insemination, on the other hand, presents a variety of legal problems involving the wife, the husband, the child, the physician, and the donor. The two most basic questions involving this procedure are: (1) Is it lawful? and (2) Is the child so conceived legitimate? There are no uniform answers to these questions and discussions of these legal aspects can be found in other sources (Artificial insemination 1957; Behrman 1975; Beck 1976).

1. INDICATIONS

The prerequisites for artificial insemination by donor (AID) include a wife who is potentially fertile with patent fallopian tubes and normal ovulatory cycles, an infertile male, and their desire to participate in the procedure. Psychologically it is important that the couple be prepared for undergoing insemination as the impact of this procedure can lead to disruption of the marriage in psychologically unstable and unprepared individuals. Those who have either ambivalent feelings or appear unable to cope with the situation should be excluded from the program or sent for professional counseling before proceeding.

Azoospermia and oligospermia with infertility of several years' duration by the husband whose wife has apparently normal fertility are the major indications for donor insemination. Marriages with Rh-negative women who have delivered one or more hydropic babies and whose husband is homozygous Rh-positive constitute an indication for insemination with a donor who is Rh-negative. Other indications include husbands with hereditary diseases that are due to the male's genes and agglutinating antibodies against spermatozoa.

Before proceeding with inseminations, the wife's fertility should be evaluated. Inseminations are expensive, time-consuming and psychologically draining and many women referred for donor insemination have been shown to have some infertility problem (Barton 1955). It is, therefore, incumbent on the physician to rule out any obvious female problem due to cervical, uterine or tubal factors which might jeopardize the success of the procedure. Ovulation can be confirmed by use of basal body temperatures in addition to either serum progesterone levels in the mid-luteal phase or an endometrial biopsy. Tubal patency can be assessed by hysterosalpinography or CO_2 insufflation; however, if pregnancy does not result within a reasonable time, it may be necessary to resort to laparoscopy in these individuals in order to rule out other causes of infertility such as pelvic inflammatory disease and pelvic endometriosis.

2. TIMING

The accurate gauging of ovulation and properly timing the inseminations is important for successful results. It is, therefore, necessary for the practitioner to study past menstrual cycles before initiation of the practice. Basal body temperature charts for three consecutive months are reviewed and the average midcycle day is calculated. Successful inseminations have been shown to occur 12 to 36 hours prior to the rise of the basal temperature (Kleegman and Kaufman 1966). It is felt that spermatozoa can maintain fertilization capabilities for 48 hours in comparison to the ovum which is throught to retain its reproductive lifespan 12 to 24 hours after ovulation, therefore best results are obtained if the inseminations are performed one to two days prior to ovulation (Behrman 1959). Delays in ovulation occur in patients undergoing inseminations (Murphy and Torrano 1963: Kohane et al. 1967), and there is a report of irregularity in the ovulatory pattern of up to 25% of the women undergoing artificial insemination (Beck 1976). Because of some cyclic variation, it is prudent to inseminate more than once per cycle. Inseminations can be performed at various time intervals to allow for the changes and shifts. Three inseminations per cycle (days 11, 13, and 15 of a 28-day cycle and days 13, 15, and 17 in a 30-day cycle) have been advocated (Guttmacher 1960); others have suggested performing one insemination 48 hours prior to the calculated rise in temperature and repeating it every other day until the shift has occurred (Beck 1974). Two inseminations per cycle around the time of ovulation, preferably scheduled on each side of the previous month's temperature shift to allow for variation, have demonstrated good results (Strickler et al. 1975).

In addition to the basal body temperature, cervical mucus spinnbarkheit and ferning and vaginal cytology can be helpful in timing ovulation (Billings et al. 1972; Cohen et al. 1956). However, irregular ovulation and anovulation necessitate regulating ovulation to increase pregnancy successes. Single i.v. injections of 20 mg of conjugated estrogens at an appropriate time have been shown to ensure the occurrence of ovulation within 24 to 48 hours of the injection in 94% of ovulatory women with irregular cycle lengths (Foldes 1972). Human chorionic gonadotropin (HCG) has been recommended in different doses (Fuchs et al. 1966; Kohane et al. 1967). Human menopausal gonadotropin has been used but is expensive and cannot be used by inexperienced individuals (Taymor and Jittivanich 1978). Use of releasing factor for insemination timing has not yielded good results (Grimes et al 1975). The most widely used agent for inducing ovulation or for changing irregular ovulatory cycles into regular ones is clomiphene citrate. A study performed several years ago utilized clomiphene on 17 ovulatory women who were undergoing AID (Klay 1976). Sixteen of these individuals became pregnant, a success rate of 94% during a mean of 1.7 treatment cycles. This high rate of success could be partially due to good timing of inseminations.

3. DONOR SELECTION FOR AID

The anonymity of the donor to the recipient couple and vice versa is very important for obvious reasons. Because of this the selection of the donor by the physician must be done in a careful manner.

There are several important factors in donor selection. Donors should be selected from pools of potentially intelligent individuals, such as college graduates, medical students, interns and residents. They should possess excellent physical health and there should be no hereditary illnesses in their family history. A negative history of drug abuse and venereal disease must also be obtained. It is preferable for the donor to have fathered children in the past to be sure of the fertility of his ejaculates even though he may have a normal semen analysis. Previously fertile individuals, however, occasionally are found to have inadequate spermatozoa for insemination, therefore it is necessary for potential donors to have a semen analysis as part of the initial evaluation. Minimal standards of greater than 40 million spermatozoa/cc with progressive motility of greater than 70% are necessary because of variations and fluctuations in all men's counts. This will help ensure fertile specimens when inseminations are performed.

The donor should have his blood typed and Rh-negative recipients should be inseminated with semen from an Rh-negative donor, if possible. The donor must be screened for venereal disease by culturing the semen for gonorrhea and obtaining a serology for syphilis.

Matching the donor with the husband is done by: (1) race, (2) eye color and (3) hair color. Because of limitations in the donor pool, it is best to use no one who is extremely short or exceptionally tall. Other characteristics such as coloring and complexion generally follow because of the coloration of eyes and hair.

4. METHODS OF INSEMINATION

There are four major methods of insemination now employed: intrauterine, (intra)cervical, cervical cap and vaginal. Often two of the methods are used simultaneously, such as intracervical and vaginal. The actual insemination is the culmination of the procedure that has involved male and female evaluations, choosing the donor, establishing an ovulatory pattern and inseminating on the proper days.

4.1. Intrauterine insemination

Intrauterine insemination involves depositing a small amount of semen (spermatozoa) directly into the endometrial cavity, thus bypassing a hostile vaginal environment and unfavorable cervical mucus. This procedure is performed only for limited indications and should almost never be utilized with AID.

4.2. Intracervical and vaginal inseminations

Intracervical insemination is performed by placing a cannula partially into the cervical canal and slowly injecting the semen. There is an overflow into the vaginal vault. In vaginal inseminations the patient is placed in slight Trendelenburg and the semen is deposited into the posterior vault. Oftentimes the speculum is adjusted in order for the cervix to bathe in the semen pool. After twenty minutes, the patient can get up from the table, dress and leave.

4.3. Cervical cap

Although there are no higher pregnancy rates for AID than with vagina intracervical inseminations, the cervical-cap technique has the advantage of allowing the patients to leave immediately, thereby not tying up rooms for long intervals. The procedure is done with one of two different designs of cervical caps. The cap without a stem has the semen placed inside the cap prior to insertion on the cervix. The upper blade of the speculum is removed and the cap is guided down the posterior blade until the cervix is reached. The cap is then pushed onto the cervix. If the cap is with a stem, then it is first put on the cervix and a small vacuum is applied. The semen is deposited through the stem afterwards. The cap can be removed after four hours or may remain on the cervix until the next morning.

5. CLINICAL SUCCESS

Donor insemination enjoys a good success rate. A potential detriment to the high conception rate is the act of mixing the semen from the husband with that of the donor. It was first demonstrated in 1960 that adding the seminal plasma from oligospermic samples with poor mobility to the spermatozoa of normal samples would severely depress the motility of the normal ejaculate (Rozin 1960). It has been shown that on occasion mixing donor and husband semen together prevented pregnancies by producing immobilization and agglutination of the donor's spermatozoa (Quinlivan and Sullivan 1977a). After stopping this practice, three of the four women became pregnant within one month. It is recommended that the husband refrain from sexual activity for two days prior to insemination because of the possibility of spermatozoal antibodies (Quinlivan and Sullivan 1977b). If the husband does, indeed, ask for mixing of the semen, this may well represent a warning that psychologically the husband has not accepted the reality of his infertility.

The pregnancy rate in donor insemination programs can be altered by silent gynecological disease. If a female recipient has no initial screening process or if the statistics include women with known gynecological problems, then the percentage success will be lower than in a normal population. This has to be kept in mind when percentages are discussed. Pregnancy rates in the literature vary in the large studies. However, cumulative pregnancy rates of approximately 90% can be achieved after six cycles – see Figure 1 (Behrman and Gosling, 1966; Chong

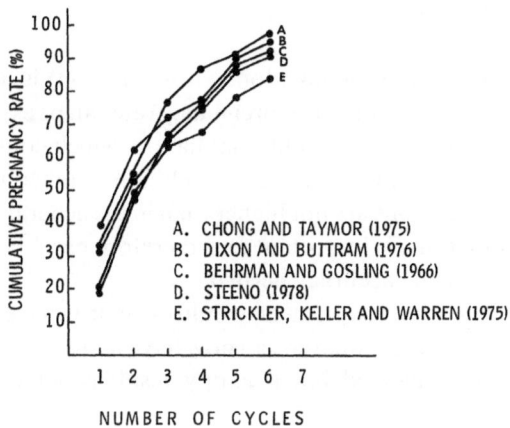

Figure 1. Cumulative pregnancy rate in donor insemination (AID).

and Taymore 1975; Dixon and Buttram 1976; Steeno 1978; Strickler et al. 1975; Sulewski et al 1978); therefore, if no pregnancy has been achieved by this time, serious thought should be given to laparoscopy (if it has not been previously performed) to explore the possibility of silent pelvic disease. Good results have been reported in large series averaging approximately 70% with participation of at least six cycles (Behrman 1959; Haman 1959; Chong and Taymor 1975; Steeno 1978; Strickler et al. 1975). Some have reported much higher rates (Klay 1976) and a few have lower rates (Dixon and Buttram 1976; Sulewski et al. 1978), but these included women with pelvic disease and utilized both fresh and frozen semen and had high dropout rates after the first few months of being in the insemination program.

Significantly, the use of frozen semen in studies has yielded lower pregnancy rates than the use of fresh semen – 73% compared to 61% (Steinberger and Smith 1973) and the number of inseminations necessary to achieve pregnancy is greater when using frozen semen. A recent study demonstrated a success rate overall of 40% (Friedman 1977), however, when correcting for 'dropouts', women who persisted for six cycles had a pregnancy rate of 61%. When women who had additional infertility problems were eliminated, a pregnancy rate of 67% was obtained, comparable to rates achieved in series utilizing fresh semen. Even though it has been claimed that the expected pregnancy rate when using frozen semen is approximately two thirds of that when using fresh semen (Behrman and Sawada 1966) the advantages may outweigh the decreased pregnancy rate.

6. CONCLUDING REMARKS

Artificial insemination heterologous (donor insemination) is a procedure that yields excellent results. A 70% or better pregnancy rate can be expected with fresh donor semen if the female has no additional factors which could affect fertility and undergoes insemination for at least six cycles. Spontaneous abortion rates and congenital malformations are not higher than in the general population. The timing of the inseminations is important and therefore basal body temperature charts are necessary for the accuracy needed.

Because of this procedure, couples who would ordinarily have to wait years for adoptive babies or go without children can now have families of their own. There are certain limitations involved but a happy result is achieved in the great majority of the time.

REFERENCES

Artificial insemination: medicine and the law. *JAMA* 163:376, 1957.
Barton M: Artificial insemination. *Stud Fertil* 7:99, 1955.
Beck WW: Artificial insemination and semen preservation *Clin Obstet Gynecol* 17:115, 1974.
Beck WW: A critical look at the legal, ethical, and technical aspects of artificial insemination. *Fertil Steril* 27:1, 1976.
Behrman SJ: Artificial insemination. *Fertil Steril* 10:248, 1959.
Behrman SJ: Artificial insemination. In: *Progress in infertility*, Behrman SJ, Kistner RW (eds), Boston, Little, Brown, 1975, p 779.
Behrman SJ, Gosling J: *Fundamentals of gynecology*, New York, Oxford University Press, 1966 (2nd ed), p 395.
Behrman SJ, Sawada Y: Heterologous and homologous inseminations with human semen frozen and stored in a liquid-nitrogen refrigerator. *Fertil Steril* 17:457, 1966.
Billings EL, Billings JJ, Brown JB, Burger HG: Symptoms and hormonal changes accompanying ovulation. *Lancet* 1:282, 1972.
Chong AP, Taymor ML: Sixteen years' experience with therapeutic donor insemination. *Fertil Steril* 26:791, 1975.
Cohen MR, Stein IR, Kaye BM: Optimal time for therapeutic insemination. *Fertil Steril* 7:141, 1956.
Dixon RE, Buttram VC: Artificial insemination using donor semen: a review of 171 cases. *Fertil Steril* 27:130, 1976.
Foldes JJ: Artificial insemination-induced ovulation with intravenous estrogens. *Int J Fertil* 17:104, 1972.
Friedman S: Artificial donor insemination with frozen human sperm. *Fertil Steril* 28:1230, 1977.
Fuchs K, Brandes JM, Paldi E: Enhancement of ovulation by choragon for successful artificial insemination. *Int J Fertil* 11:211, 1966.
Goss DA: Current status of artificial insemination with donor semen. *Am J Obstet Gynecol* 122:246, 1975.
Grimes EM, Taymor ML, Thomson IE: Induction of timed ovulation with synthetic luteinizing hormone-releasing hormone in women undergoing insemination therapy. *Fertil Steril* 26:277, 1975.
Guttmacher AF: The role of artificial insemination in the treatment of sterility. *Obstet Gynecol Survey* 15:767, 1960.
Haman JO: Therapeutic donor insemination: a review of 440 cases. *Calif Med* 90:130, 1959.

Klay LJ: Clomiphene-regulated ovulation for donor artificial insemination. *Fertil Steril* 27:383, 1976.

Kleegman S, Amelar RD, Sherman JK, Hirschhorn K, Pilpel H: Artificial donor insemination (round table). *Med. Aspects Human Sexuality* 4:85, 1970.

Kleegman SJ, Kaufman SA: *Infertility in women.* Oxford, Blackwell, 1966.

Kohane ES, Sharf M, Kreminsky T: The use of HCG in delayed ovulation during artificial insemination. *Fertil Steril* 18:593, 1967.

Murphy DP, Torrano EF: The day of conception: a study of 48 women having two or more conceptions by donor insemination. *Fertil Steril* 14:410, 1963.

Quinlivan WLG, Sullivan H: The immunologic effects of husband's semen on donor spermatozoa during mixed insemination. *Fertil Steril* 28:448, 1977a.

Quinlivan WLG, Sullivan H: Spermatozoal antibodies in human seminal plasma as a cause of failed artificial insemination. *Fertil Steril* 28:1082, 1977b.

Rohleder H: *Test tube babies*, New York, Vantage, 1943.

Rozin S: Studies on seminal plasma I: the role of seminal plasma in motility of spermatozoa. *Fertil Steril* 11:278, 1960.

Shields FE: Artificial insemination as related to female. *Fertil Steril* 1:271, 1950.

Steeno O: Cervical cap technique of insemination. Presented at the first international symposium on AIH and male subfertility, Bordeaux, 1978.

Steinberger E, Smith KD: Artificial insemination with fresh or frozen semen. *JAMA* 223:778, 1973.

Strickler RC, Keller DW, Warren JC: Artificial insemination with fresh donor semen. *New Eng J Med* 293:848, 1975.

Sulewski JM, Eisenberg F, Steinger VG: A longitudinal analysis of artificial insemination with donor semen. *Fertil Steril* 29:527, 1978.

Taymor ML, Jittivanich B: Ovulation regulation with HMG for artificial insemination. Presented at the first international symposium on AIH and male subfertility, Bordeaux, 1978.

18. ARTIFICIAL INSEMINATION WITH FRESH DONOR SEMEN

P.E.R. RHEMREV, C.C.A. DE NOOYER and W.A.A. VAN OS

INTRODUCTION

The recent and rapid decline in adoptable infants in the Netherlands has brought about an increase in the use of artificial insemination, and changing cultural views have influenced the question of the use of donor semen. Women who feel themselves capable of childbearing prefer to mother their own natural children; their infertile husbands understand this and feel that it is preferable for these children to be brought up by at least one natural parent. Thus, if there is a stable marriage and a deep desire to have children AID can be started. The only important fact is that according to Dutch law the husband must recognize the future child as his legal child. We do not demand prior psychological evaluation of the future parents, for the value of this remains in our opinion unclear.

Before starting the AID procedure the following must be fulfilled:
1. Both husband and wife must ask 'spontaneously' for AID;
2. The husband must have been proved infertile (mostly azoospermia);
3. The wife must have been proved fertile.

We only strongly discourage couples from undergoing AID in cases of age nearing 40. We also advise the couple not to announce their intentions to family or friends.

2. PATIENTS

Fertility evaluation of the woman has to be performed extensively by the use of basal body temperature charts for a minimum of three months (establishment of length of menstrual cycle - see Table 1), endometrial biopsy, and hysterography. Women with a so-called short post-ovulation period, showing a short period of temperature rise were excluded from this investigation also because of a great chance of being infertile. Again, the husband must be of proven infertility (Table 2) because, in cases of sexual deviation, AID is contraindicated even by way of treatment.

Table 1. Menstrual cycles (regular) of 142 women treated with AID.

Length of cycle (days)	Number of women
26	12
28	82
30	22
32	14
34	10
36	2

Table 2. Husbands with proven infertility (142).

Cause	Number	Remarks
Azoospermia	83	
Oligospermia	55	Less than 10×10^6 per millilitre with infertility of long duration
Klinefelter's syndrome	3	All had azoospermia
Vasectomized	1	Because of genetic disease

3. DONORS

Donors are selected by physical examination and were screened anamnestically for genetic diseases. Their semen must be of proven fertility and/or be examined microscopically; it must fulfill normal standards of fertile semen.

Since no child is an exact portrait of his parents it is unnecessary to attempt to match the donor exactly to the husband. In our series, blood, rhesus, eye color, and general racial characteristics, including European and Mediterranean categories, were the only ones matched. The babies born so far have all been accepted by their parents and, more importantly, by their legal fathers. Because of the fact that all donors were students of ages between 20 and 25 years, no investigations were done into social backgrounds, special talents, or indeed into rare hereditary diseases, because these are unlikely to be discovered in apparently healthy young men. No screening for VD was done since this is uncommon in medical students and there is no guarantee that a young man who is free from infection at the first screening will not contract the disease later.

4. TECHNIQUE

Fresh semen was used entirely because of our (still) bad results with frozen semen. The semen specimens were delivered about an hour before the recipients

arrived and were placed in an incubator. The donors and recipients were unknown to each other. After evaluation of basal body temperature graph the
moment of ovulation was diagnosed. During this period a small fraction of
cervical mucus was examined for color, viscosity, ferning, and cellularity. A
Kurzrok-Miller in vitro test with available semen with cervical mucus was
performed. When tests had satisfactory results the AID procedure was performed. About 2-3 ml of fresh semen was placed in a small plastic cup adjusted
to the cervix by a slight vacuum. Thus, a close contact with the cervical area was
obtained as long as the cup remained in situ. After four hours the cup was
removed by the woman herself without doctors' help.

Two days after the insemination procedure the basal body temperature graph
was analysed again. If no rise of temperature was noticed and all cervical factors
showed a preovulatory pattern as described earlier the insemination procedure
was started again. Using this undoubtedly time-consuming method it was possible to limit the insemination procedure to twice per menstrual cycle only.
Friberg (1974) has already described the adverse effect of seminal plasma from
one man to spermatozoa from another man, so we advised the woman not to
have intercourse within three days of the expected rise in basal body temperature
(Quinlivan 1977), since even in cases of oligospermia, intercourse prior to insemination may render added donor semen immobile because of spermatozoal
antibodies.

5. RESULTS

The 142 women underwent the AID procedure twice during a menstrual cycle.
After a six-month period of inseminations 56 (40%) of the recipients became
pregnant; after twelve months a total of 99 (71%) had become pregnant. The
remaining unsuccessful women were treated with epinestrol preovulatory. From
this group six became pregnant after a treatment of six months; two became
pregnant three months later, after treatment with Epinestrol and Clomiphene
citrates.

At the end, 35 women remained infertile after 24 months of insemination
with or without therapy. These 35 underwent a laparoscopy and a semen antibody investigation. No anatomical variations of internal genitals were seen; nor
were antibodies diagnosed. The cervical area showed no local deviations by
Papanicolaou smears or bacterial cultures.

From the 56 women who became pregnant after a period of six months of
insemination two pregnancies ended in a spontaneous abortion and one in a
stillbirth due to a severe toxemia of pregnancy.

From the 43 remaining women who became pregnant between a period of six
and twelve months of insemination, three pregnancies ended in a spontaneous

abortion and one woman gave birth to a girl with a deformation of the right hand. One of the epinestrol and clomiphene citrate induced pregnancies needed a curettage because of a spontaneous abortion after eight weeks of pregnancy. One hundred women gave birth to a baby and one had a stillbirth. From these 101 babies born to inseminated women, there have been 58 girls and 43 boys. The stillbirth baby was a female.

6. CONCLUSION

Approximately 75% of 142 women artificially inseminated with fresh donor semen had a good result, as far as a positive pregnancy test counts. We are aware that our results are lower when compared with Newill (1976) and Koren (1976); their figures of success are 85% and 80% respectively. But on the other side approximating the numbers given by Goldenberg (75%) we are not able to find a satisfactory explanation for this discrepancy, but on the other hand a similar success rate (75%) was reported by Goldenberg (1977). Neither can we give an explanation as to the preponderance of girls in our results, which are in contrast to some published figures for AID (Seymour 1941; Steinberger 1973). The reason for the infertility of 25% of the recipients can not yet be answered, but it may be due to an unnoticed corpus luteum deficiency (Campana 1976), even though we treated all those 35 unsuccessful women with clomiphene citrate. Five-percent spontaneous abortions is an acceptable percentage, especially when compared with other investigators, such as the 10-13% found by Gigon (1977). We can at least conclude that AID is a useful and an increasingly acceptable technique for bringing children into those childless families who are plagued by male infertility.

7. SUMMARY

The aim of this investigation was to minimize artificial insemination to two inseminations, using fresh semen, per menstrual cycle. Application of semen was performed by a cervical cap. One hundred and forty-two women with treated regular menstrual cycles and ovulations were treated. The indication for artificial insemination with donor semen (AID) was mostly azoospermia of the husband. Fifty-six (40%) of the treated women had become pregnant after a period of six months. After twelve months a total of 99 (71%) women were pregnant. The remaining 43 women were treated with epinestrol preovulatory. After six months of insemination six women became pregnant and at least two further pregnancies occurred after treatment with epinestrol and clomiphene citrate.

REFERENCES

Campana A: Abort Frequenz und Abort Ursachen bei Schwangerschaften nach Teterologen Insemi-
    nationen. *Geburtsh Frauenheilk* 36:421, 1976.
Friberg J: Immunological studies on human sperm-agglutinating seminal fluid. *Acta Obstet Gynecol
    Scand* 53 (suppl):56, 1974.
Goldenberg RL: AID *J Reprod Med* 18:149, 1977.
Newill, P: AID: a review of 200 cases. *Br J Urol* 48:139, 1976.
Quinlivan WLG: Spermatozoal antibodies in human seminal plasma as a cause of failed AID *Fertil
    Steril* 28:1082, 1977.
Seymour FI: AID: present status in the US as shown by recent survey. *JAMA* 116:2747, 1941.
Steinberger E: AID with fresh or frozen semen. *JAMA* 223:778, 1973.

19. PSYCHOLOGICAL AND SEXUAL PROBLEMS OF AIH

A. MATTEI, A.M. BOLCIONI-AUTARD, M.C. BOUHABEN-SITRI
and R. ROULIER

1. SEXUAL PROBLEMS LEADING TO AIH

Irrespective of the nature of the dysfunction, it is necessary to specify the diagnosis before undertaking any type of AIH treatment. Three questions should be considered:

1. Should sexological therapy be sought and particularly a brief behavioral therapy?

2. Is AIH considered by the couple as an aid or a recognition by the physician of an incurable condition?

3. Is the trouble manageable or is a personality disorder of either partner apparent, thus making child-raising difficult?

2. PSYCHOLOGICAL CONSEQUENCES OF AIH IN THE THERAPY OF CONJUGAL STERILITY

Mrs. D: We had thought of AIH even before it was proposed to us. We were happy to start the therapy, as it presented new hope. We thought we would have an extra chance by the introduction in the cervix of split ejaculate. We became less enthusiastic after several menstrual cycles. I was always hopeful, but slowly became discouraged. It became more and more difficult to come to the center – for my husband, who was distracted in his work and who once, after six or seven inseminations during one cycle, could not ejaculate – for me, living each month to the rhythm of ovulation and menstrual period. I was more anxious than before of my impending periods because I was more hopeful. There are both good times and bad times in our sex life without any particular reason. At the moment of artificial insemination, I felt stripped of my sex and my body. I considered it was a medical act and I leant my body to it. I felt my sex organs no longer existed, that they were only genital organs. All this had repercussions on our sex life. Little by little, our relations became less frequent, less satisfying. They were better just before my periods. When my period came, I was in tears.

Mr. D: Your body became a machine, noticed by your doctor and yourself. The curve became more important. It worked well or not at all. For my part, there was a fear of not being able to ejaculate. We have not felt that artificial insemination is a miracle method. It was important to be informed of the small chance of success so as not to become too optimistic. We would have asked to be treated, anyway, for at least three menstrual cycles. It would have been an error on our part not to have done it. We would not have been satisfied if we had not tried it. We would have preferred it if they had fixed a delay rather than saying 'It might succeed.' Eight months is too long. Three months would have been enough. We were well received and that counts a lot.

3. CLINICAL ASPECTS

The couple deciding on AIH is already traumatized from their past explorations and treatments of their sterility. Optimism and discouragement alternated during treatment modification and at onset of menstruation. Several problems may arise: (1) the significance of a married couple without children; (2) the significance of children, of life, of death; (3) the present status of the couple could be questioned; (4) the sex life of the married couple is influenced by the thermogenic shift and the onset of menstruation; and (5) even the notion of virility and femininity can be questioned.

Artificial insemination, therefore, seems to be the last resort, after which there is only sterility, helplessness, and grief. It also appears to be a miracle method in the treatment of male hypofertility, sometimes confused with artificial fecundity.

The method of AIH alters the sex life as follows: (1) patient observation of her basal body temperature chart; (2) physician observation of the chart and cervical mucus; (3) prohibited sexual relations during ovulation; (4) with the obligation of split ejaculation, fear of failure, and therefore, feeling of guilt towards the partner; and (5) replacement of an inefficient conjugal relationship by another involving a third person which might become successful.

These disturbances extend beyond married life and can affect the professional and social life of the couple, such as absence from work for several days, asking for permission to be absent, and explaining the treatment to superiors and colleagues.

The inconveniences are more severe in the case of male hypofertility than when artificial insemination is indicated by a female problem. Male procreative capacity is questioned and therefore the chances of success are fewer.

A comparison can be made with the psychological problems raised by AID. The difference appears to be fundamental: the acceptance of using donor sperm presupposes that the husband has accepted his problem of sterility and that the couple has disassociated the biological and the sociological aspects of paternity. This acceptance requires a long psychological adjustment during which time psychological assistance and/or counselling is beneficial. Artificial insemination is not presented as a miracle treatment, but rather as a palliative treatment. Finally, the utilization of good-quality sperm permits a higher success rate.

In the presence of male hypofertility, many couples foresee a trial of AIH (even on a short-term basis, as in the case we reported) prior to resorting to AID. Others desire a mixture of their sperm with that of a donor, a method justifiably challenged by most researchers. Our goal is not to dramatize the situation concerning couples desiring AIH, but rather to draw attention to the psychological factors which inhibit couples and to recognize our present rates of success.

Prevention of difficulties are possible if, before starting therapy, counselling takes place in order to evaluate the couple's sexual and psychological status, to inform them of the method of therapy, of the chances of success and also the risks of disturbing the couple's sex life, and to fix a reasonable number of cycles at the end of which, if necessary, an AID could be undertaken. During therapy, the couple should be informed regularly of the treatment procedures and their reaction should be noted.

4. CONCLUSION

The secondary psychological and sexual problems of AIH are due to the fact that couples, weakened by a long period of sterility, continuing their struggle optimistically, are offered yet another trying method of therapy, for which the success rate has been low.

20. AIH FOR SEXUAL INADEQUACY

J. TIGNOL

1. INTRODUCTION

AIH constitutes the most tasteful and most easily acceptable solution for certain male sterilities due to organic causes. With this method, one can obtain an infant of the couple and not an 'infant of another' as with AID. Thus, one can be tempted to use it in the cases of sterility due to a sexual dysfunction of psychological origin.

2. SEXUAL PROBLEMS CAN LEAD TO STERILITY OF A COUPLE

2.1. Description of problems

Problems may be divided into two categories: unconsummated marriage and anejaculation.

2.1.1. Unconsummated marriage. Unconsummated marriage is classically described as being due both to female and male causes, frequently forming a problem of the couple (Pasini 1971, 1978). Female problems include dyspareunia and vaginismus. When the only concern is fertility and the desire to have a child, dyspareunia is not an obstacle. The prognosis is excellent (>90%) for vaginismus when treated with brief psychotherapy. Since there is no significant relationship between frigidity and sterility, it seems completely unreasonable to propose AIH in cases where there is only female sexual dysfunction. On the other hand, all female sexual dysfunction and particularly dyspareunia and vaginismus, will considerably aggravate any male sexual dysfunction responsible for the unconsummated marriage. In the male, erectile dysfunction (impotence) or ultra-premature ejaculation (ante portas) can either alone, or more frequently associated, prevent penetration. The association or frequently the alternation of these two dysfunctions in the same patients, enables us to study them as one sexual dysfunction. This makes up a homogenous group of cases of sterility. From a purely technical viewpoint, it is easy to envisage the collection of sperm to perform AIH with a fertile partner.

2.1.2. Anejaculation. Anejaculation permits penetration of the partner, but similar to the previous group, intravaginal ejaculation never occurs. There are two subgroups: patients who can never ejaculate while awake, and present only pollutions; and patients who can ejaculate while awake, either by masturbating or having their partner stimulate them to ejaculate outside the vagina – cases where the vagina is always taboo for ejaculation. For the latter patients, masturbation is efficient for the collection of sperm. However, in the first group, the collection of sperm during nocturnal pollutions is acrobatic (condom without any spermicidal agent). Certain vibrators seem to be efficient to 'force' an ejaculation even in the absence of erection, to collect sperm for an AIH. We will see that these two subgroups seem very different concerning their psychic functioning and their prognosis of the treatment.

2.2. Psychological considerations

Sexual dysfunction is a symptom which results from a complex, unconscious intrapsychic conflict. This symptom is a defense for the subject even though he is bothered by it. It is considered in dynamic psychopathology that one should not try to suppress a symptom brutally or to change it under penalty of seeing it get worse or simply change form. These blunt statements are often filled with nuances.

It is more important to know that men, not having consummated their marriages are more often 'emotionally immature', namely, that they have a purely neurotic problem in relation to the Oedipal complex, a large emotional dependence upon their love object, in this case, their wife. The wife usually has a sexual and psychological dysfunction in some way complementary to the husband's. One is almost always surprised at the misinterpretation by the couple of the most elementary sexual matters. The pathology of the couple reinforces the pathology of the individual in the absence of treatment. These men feel worthless and unconfident by their inability to penetrate (Held 1968).

The patients appear differently in a case of anejaculation. They do not seem to suffer from their problem. If they were not pushed by their wife and her desire to have a child, they would not seek medical advice. It is true that in relation to standard masculine values, the anejaculator is able to 'save face' remarkably well. Only his wife is not fooled; she feels frustrated despite the possibility of prolonged lovemaking. If the symptom of anejaculation represents a defense at the anal level (according to psychoanalytic terminology), the personality structure of the patient does not necessarily correlate to obsessional neurosis nor to an anal character. An individual psychodynamic evaluation is necessary for each patient. It is hoped to draw dynamic indications of the symptom itself. It seems that the classic anejaculators, those that can only ejaculate while sleeping or never, are neurotic in the broad sense of the term: their conflicts are kept to themselves; they have solid emotional ties with their wives and a relation without perversity. One can compare them to the cases of anejaculators 'incomplete', who can ejaculate by masturbating and who present more of a pathological character. They project their internal conflicts on their surroundings and have a moderately perverse relation with their partner. If this is verified by a greater number of cases than mine, this distinction will be important because it has a certain prognostic value. One knows that a neurotic personality is more apt to benefit from psychotherapy than one who presents a pathological character.

2.3. Psychotherapeutic treatment

2.3.1. Methods. Psychoanalysis (therapy dealing with personality problems and not with sexual problems) will not be discussed here. Any sexual problems that improve are treated secondarily to personal problems. Patients asking for AIH are far from asking for psychoanalysis. Brief dynamic psychotherapy on the other hand constitutes in most of the cases an adequate treatment. Often these psychotherapies use as support a supplementary method, for example auto- genous relaxation training or narcoanalysis or different behavioral techniques. These can be directed toward the individual but more often are oriented for the couple.

2.3.2. Results. The effectiveness of these methods is proven and Held (1968) affirms that the indication of psychoanalytic psychotherapy is imperative and published a case of a cure from only one session. Masters and Johnson (1971) cured 14 of the 17 cases. Gellman and Gellman (1978) reported 7 successes out of 12 patients who had agreed to undergo a treatment. In four of my cases treated by a brief psychotherapy, in sessions far apart, I have had three successes and one interruption of treatment. This was a couple that was without ejaculation for 18 years.

The prognosis of ultra-premature ejaculation is similar to that of impotence, with which it is often associated; it does not have the same prognosis as that of ordinary premature ejaculation, which is $>90\%$. Sexological statistics (Kaplan 1974) are variable in the form of the problem and the selection of cases. Held (1968) cured 8 out of 10 cases of impotence, but·he is a very good psycho- therapist. Pasini's results (1971) were successful in 12 out of 15 couples that he treated for non-consummated marriages. Only 5 of these couples consulted him to have a child, the other 10 for sexual problems. In most patients the desire for sexual fulfillment is greater than the wish to procreate, which is fairly natural. The motive for the consultation did not have any influence on the prognosis of the brief psychotherapy of the couple which was done by Pasini.

2.3.3. Significance. The significance of the psychotherapeutic cure of the symp- tom is variable. In the good cases, there is a slight modification of the psychic functioning of the subject, who put back into his relationship with the spouse, becomes durable and at best permits an autonomous progression after the psychotherapy. One has obtained more than a simple disappearance of the symptom. In other cases, the subject becomes cured of his symptoms to avoid any profound changes, to escape from being cured of his disease. Therefore one can expect a relapse, another symptom, or a reinforcement of character troubles. It is difficult for the psychotherapist to be satisfied with this result, but there is still the possibility of undertaking the treatment again.

In general, sterility by sexual dysfunction can be 'cured' in one-half to two-thirds of the cases by a brief psychotherapy of the couple. This method of treatment has the advantage of permitting a natural conception leading to psychological well-being for the two partners.

3. AIH FOR SEXUAL PROBLEMS OF PSYCHOLOGICAL ORIGIN

3.1. The request for AIH

3.1.1. Frequency. The propagation of sexological information, and more recently, information on AIH for the public and for the doctors has changed from year to year the number of demanding couples and the form of their demand. It is the sperm banks that make the anejaculators appear. Before this, medical advice was sought so rarely that one thought this was a rare pathology. Pasini's five couples, who consulted a sexologist in 1971 to have a child, would probably have gone first to see a gynecologist or an andrologist for an AIH in 1978. Since 1971, I have seen more and more anejaculators, and in the last year three couples have initially demanded an AIH; one was an anejaculator and two were non-consummated marriages. According to Delafontaine (1978), 'the sexological indications of AIH merit a preliminary interview with a psychiatrist or at least a reflection by the inseminator'. If the indication of AIH for sexological problems is allowed with few reservations, one can foresee a notable increase in the demand for insemination for sexual dysfunction.

3.1.2. Significance. The reluctance provoked, in most people, no matter what their cultural level, in contemplating the prospect of a psychological treatment is great. Lack of information, pressure from other people, and medical prejudices are to blame, but there are also resistances of the patient, reinforcing the individual's unconscious, which rule over his sorting of information, over the choice of the consulting doctor. One must remember that the interior psychological phenomena of the couple are first a factor of amplification of the resistances. Once the treatment is started, the same phenomenon amplifies the favorable changes. Each partner is afraid of unmasking his complaints against the other or his erotic fantasies. Guilty thoughts or desires or a feeling of guilt without a conscious motive can create a fear of losing the other. Here AIH seems very secure: it does not involve pathological equilibrium of the couple. The birth of the child does not obliterate this disequilibrium nor the very probable persistence of the sexual dysfunction and pathology of the couple.

3.2. The response of the inseminating doctor

The practice of AIH for sexual problems without initially trying to treat the dysfunction can be attributed to two factors.
1. The lack of knowledge of the possibilities of psychotherapy for sexual trouble, which goes from simple lack of information to prejudices against psychoanalysis, psychology or psychiatry;
2. The temptation to use a new technique that allows the doctor, in keeping with current medical ideology, to respond directly and intelligently to the demand. The pressure of the demand to have a child can also reinforce this temptation.

4. DISCUSSION OF THE EVENTUAL INDICATIONS FOR AIH FOR STERILITY DUE TO SEXUAL PROBLEMS

The indications for insemination always raise passionate discussions.

4 1 Arguments for immediate AIH

The desire of the couple and the inseminating doctor can be evoked to practice an AIH without any other preliminary treatment in a case of sterility due to sexual problems. The liberty of people could also be an argument. This liberty has legal limits when it is a question of adopting a child, but medical limits only for some in the indication of AID.

One can also argue in favor of AIH from certain developments of psychoanalytic theory. The patients with 'neurosis of behaviour' are incapable of controlling their interior conflicts by means of internal mental operation. They do not find any escape from their conflicts except in acting them out in their life (projection of these conflicts on the exterior world, the search for a security object at any price with the penalty of decompensated depression or a psychosomatic illness) in a disordered manner and often with little benefit. These patients are not very good candidates for psychotherapeutic treatment. One can imagine that the diagnosis of such a personality structure would make one prefer an immediate AIH over a possible failure of psychotherapy.

4.2. Arguments against an immediate AIH

All of the arguments in favor of psychotherapy for sexual dysfunction are arguments against AIH. AIH has several consequences:

1. The continuation of the sexual problem does not change very much for the anejaculator as long as his wife does not only take care of the child. On the other hand a person with impotence will have his condition aggravated by AIH when paternity brings along with it illusion and inferiority.

2. It brings about the reinforcement of the resistance to psychotherapy, or more likely, the disappearance of the need for treatment of the wife, who has satisfied her desire for a child.

3. There is a pejorative influence on the development of the child, raised by a neurotic couple, neurotic to the point of presenting a symptom as important as that of anejaculation, and especially an unconsummated marriage. Fortunately for them, a certificate of mental health is not demanded from either partner to have children. On the other hand, there are couples much sicker than our AIH demanders who procreate without any obstacles of future mental and social handicaps. One should anyway think before enabling a couple to have a child by a medical procedure if one knows this couple presents an evident neurosis.

Further there are couples in whom the sexual symptom is not the result of neurotic malfunctioning but is the result of a psychotic personality or a border-line case not yet decompensated. The treatment of the sexual problem is counterindicated under penalty of serious decompensation (Pasini 1971; Labrousse 1978). AIH is also obviously counterindicated in these cases.

4.3. AIH after failure of psychotherapy for sexual dysfunction

Failure of psychotherapy occurs among the couples that are most psychologically disturbed. It would therefore seem logical not to enable them to have a child by AIH, but only a multidisciplinary study of the indications for AIH and the follow-up of the AIH can make things clear to us in an acceptable manner. It is necessary to get study groups together to unite inseminating doctors who do not deny the psychic effect and psychotherapeutic specialists who do not have any anti-medical prejudices. On the condition that these people know each other, are interested in this work, and do not have any territorial conflicts between them, their collaboration would have a chance to be fruitful for the patient and for scientific knowledge.

5. CONCLUSION

To practice an AIH for sterility due to sexual dysfunction seems disputable. The first treatment in these cases is that of the sexual dysfunction. In case of failure the indication for AIH must be studied in a multidisciplinary research group. Codification of these indications necessitates further study.

REFERENCES

Cohen J: *Les Stérilités et hypofertilités masculines*, Paris, Masson, 1972, p 214 (2nd ed).
Delafontaine D: *L'insémination artificielle: définition. indications, programmation, réalisation, technique et résultats. Contraception-Fertilité-Sexualité*. 6 (8):511, 1978.
Friedmand LJ: *Virgin wives*. London, Tavistock, 1962.
Geboes K, Steeno O, DeMoor P: Primary anejaculation: diagnosis and therapy. *Fertil Steril* 26 (10:1018), 1975.
Gellman R, Gellman C: Contribution à l'étude de l'absence d'éjaculation. *Cahiers de Sexologie Clinique* 4 (20):183, 1978.
Held RR: *Psychothérapie et psychanalyse*, Paris, Payot, 1968.
Kaplan HS: *The new sex therapy*, London, Baillère-Tindall, 1974.
Labrousse D: La place du psychiatre dans la gynécologie. *Bordeaux Medical* 11 (16):1441, 1978.
Marty P: *Les mouvements individuels de vie et de mort*, Payot, Paris, 1976.
Masters WH, Johnson VC: *Les Mésententes sexuelles*, Paris, Laffont, 1971.
Measson-Chevret M: Le vécu de l'insémination artificielle. Thèse médecine, Lyon 89, 1977, summary in: L'insémination artificielle avec donneur Vrylon R, *Nouv Presse Méd* 7 (10):857, 1978.
Michel-Wolfromm H: *Cette chose-là*. Paris, Grasset, 1970.
Nijs P: Aspects psychosomatiques de l'insémination artificielle. *Cahiers de Sexologie Clinique* 3:261, 1976.
Pasini W: Les mariages non consommés, problème de couple. *Médecine et Hygiène* 29:2035, 1971.
Pasini W: Cause psicologiche della sterilità e loro terapia. *Sessuologia* 1:76, 1978.
Schellen TMCM: Induction of ejaculation by electrovibration. *Fertil Steril* 19 (4):566, 1968.
Sobrero AS, Stearns HE, Blair JH: Technic for the induction of ejaculation in humans. *Fertil Steril* 16 (6):765, 1965.

21. LEGAL AND ETHICAL ASPECTS OF ARTIFICIAL INSEMINATION

H. AMIRIKIA and J. H. BOOKER

1. INTRODUCTION

It is estimated that in the US 10-15% of married couples are infertile (Behrman and Kistner 1968). The portion of infertility cases due to the male factor runs from 10-50% (Kraus and Quinn 1977) with an average of 35% (Kraus 1976) of all cases being due to the male. Since the legalization of abortion in the US the number of babies available for adoption has decreased, while the public's awareness of artificial insemination with donor sperm (AID) has increased. As a result the demand for artificial insemination has grown in all Western countries (primarily the US). It has, in fact, been accepted as the new modality in the management of couples desiring children where the male is infertile. It is estimated that between 6,000 and 10,000 AID children are born in the US each year (Curie-Cohen et al. 1979). However many unresolved legal questions related to AID exist.

Artificial insemination with donor sperm can be a very effective method of producing a pregnancy where the husband is infertile. Psychological assessment is at present the most difficult factor in estimating the benefits of this technique. Therefore the medical practitioner must investigate all psychological elements in great depth.

We are living in an era in which it is becoming increasingly fashionable for academics and practitioners to engage in interdisciplinary activities and studies. One such combination incorporates law and biology, within which is included the subject of artificial insemination. It is apparent that some legal guidelines must be instituted to define the rights and liabilities of all parties involved: the parents, donor, doctor, and child.

Several aspects of this issue must be considered: Who may perform the procedure? What type of consent is required? What parameters exist for the selection of a donor? What potential for future liability exists? What is the legal identity of the offspring?

2. WHO CAN PERFORM AID?

The practice of AID has been restricted to physicians. Curiously the state of Kansas does not limit the performance of artificial insemination to physicians; there presumably anyone can legally perform the technique. Additional information as to who can perform AID is contained in the section on state legislation.

3. INFORMED CONSENT

A major problem in AID is the determination of the meaning of 'informed, voluntary, and competent consent.' Until the legal ambiguities are resolved by statute to protect the rights of all parties who are involved in AID, including the administering physicians and their insurers, a consent agreement should be implemented to protect them from liability.

The physician who performs the artificial insemination should request both the husband and wife to sign a consent form stating that they understand the concept of AID and that they release the physician from any legal liability should the child suffer a disability, abnormality, or congenital defect or not be born with all the mental and physical characteristics expected by either the husband or wife.

AID exposes its participants to a multiplicity of emotional factors (Macourt and Jones 1977). The husband must have complete acceptance of his own sterility; have a strong desire to participate in and allow his wife the experience of childbirth; have no feelings of hostility or resentment towards the child; and be willing to accept the child as his own. The wife must have no hostility or resentment towards her husband. The couple must have no negative moral or social attitudes towards the AID. Their marriage must be stable, and communication between the partners must be good, particularly in regard to the AID.

Moral objections to artificial insemination have come mainly from organized religion. The majority of Catholic theological opinion opposes not only AID but also artificial insemination with the husband's sperm (AIH). The Lutheran and Jewish Orthodox faiths also oppose both forms of artificial insemination and only under a situation of extreme need does rabbinic opinion permit AID; therefore individual cases must be presented to rabbinic authority before the AID is performed (Amelar et al. 1977). Most other Christian religions do not oppose artificial insemination in principle. Islamic opinion strongly opposes the practice of AID.

In 1960 a lay committee reported on artificial insemination in the United Kingdom. They designated that the practice of AID is an undesirable and immoral liberty comparable to fornication and adultery and that its practice should be strongly discouraged. One of the issues often brought up by opponents

of AID is that of innocent incest when two offspring of the same donor marry or
form a sexual relationship (Beck 1976). The statistical probability of such incest
occurring is extremely low and can be regulated by a limit being set by law on the
number of times that a given donor can be used.

4. SELECTION OF A DONOR

The question of who will serve as a donor of sperm has implications beyond strict
medical concerns. The social and political implications of the donor process raise
interesting questions which are also inferred from the potential use of AID in
genetic engineering.

New York City has regulated the practice of donor selection through its
Health Code since 1948. The ordinance provides that no donor shall have 'any
disease or defect known to be transmissible by the genes.' It also requires blood
grouping and Rh typing of donors.

5. LIABILITY

Potential liability in AID is similar to that in other areas of law as it pertains
to medicine and the family. Up to this point there have been no reported court
cases based either on medical malpractice or the theory of wrongful life. This is
probably due to the shroud of secrecy surrounding the practice of AID and the
usual presumption of legitimacy of a child born during wedlock. It is important
to remember that the legal system in the US has not always looked with favor
upon AID. It is also important to bear in mind that the response of the law has
been inconsistent and sometimes contradictory, which makes it very difficult
to predict with any amount of certainty how any specific case will be handled.
Three main sources exist for finding answers: court cases, state legislatures, and
proposed uniform legislation.

In most states the legal paternity can be attributed to either the husband or
the donor. The legal responsibility of the physician performing the AID, in
regard to paternity, remains unclear. In fact in the cases that have been ad-
judicated there has been little problem in establishing paternity with the husband
as long as there is informed consent by both partners.

Another problem that may arise for the obstetrician is that of whose name to
enter on the birth certificate as the father. Is the physician who performed the
AID guilty of fraud by executing a birth certificate while withholding the information that the mother's husband is not the natural father of the child? To
avoid possible liability the physician who performed the insemination may, for
delivery, refer the patient to another physician who is unaware of how the child

was conceived (Frankel 1974; Goldenberg and White 1977). Of course this raises a serious question of medical ethics.

6. LEGAL IDENTITY OF THE CHILD

The fundamental problem confronting the US legal system where AID is concerned has been the legal identity of the child conceived by AID, and the effect of this identity upon the donor of sperm, the mother, the husband, the physician, and the institution providing the insemination.

A marital union has been accepted as the appropriate context for conception, delivery, and upbringing of a child. In the Anglo-American legal system legitimate children possess the power to inherit from both their father and mother since the husband of the wife is the father of the child. Legitimate children have the right to claim the necessities of life from their biological parents and, likewise, the parents of legitimate offspring are accorded significant areas of decision-making affecting the rearing of their children. Illegitimacy has been regarded unfavorably. In conception with artificial insemination, since the husband of the mother is not the biological father of the child, the question of legitimacy remains an issue of primary importance.

The effect of AID children on the family unit is said to compare favorably with that of adopted children. Among several hundred couples there was no case in which AID caused any psychological problem to the couple. Marriage on the whole was said to improve after the AID and couples reported increased satisfaction with their marriage. If desire for further children was felt, willingness to undergo AID again was expressed. Occasional adverse emotional reactions following the birth of an AID child which have disturbed marital relations have been reported. In one report the woman became infatuated with the unknown donor and changed her attitude towards her husband even to the extent of leaving him.

The legal status of AID children is uncertain (Rosenberg 1968). Are they legitimate? Do they have the same legal rights as biological children of both parents? Do they have the same legal rights as adopted children? What are their rights to inheritance, support and custody? But where consent to the technique of AID is expressed by both parents there is little justification for the courts to deny legitimacy and its incidental rights to children born as a result (Carr 1973).

7. STATE LEGISLATION

Seven state legislatures have enacted legislation regarding AID: Georgia, Oklahoma, Kansas, California, North Carolina, Maryland and Arkansas (Healey

1976). Oklahoma and Kansas have statutes containing explicit information on the legality of the performance of AID. In the remaining five states such information appears to be implicit.

Who can perform AID? Georgia and Oklahoma have answered this question by stating that only those who are licensed to practice medicine can perform AID. In Kansas artificial insemination can be performed by any person duly authorized to practice medicine at the request of and with consent in writing from the husband and wife desiring the utilization of the technique for the purpose of conceiving a child or children. Any child or children born as a result of this conception shall be considered by law in all respects as legitimate and naturally conceived. The propriety of permitting persons other than physicians to perform AID is questionable, since the general public could be subjected to the ineptitude of 'cut-rate' practitioners whose activities would be most difficult to supervise and regulate. Conceivably even mail-ordering of human sperm complete with 'do-it-yourself' instructions and supplies would not be prohibited by statute.

In Georgia the physician or surgeon is relieved of civil liability to the husband and wife for any child conceived by artificial insemination or the results providing he obtains written consent. However this authorization shall not relieve any physician or surgeon from his negligent administration or performance of artificial insemination.

Six states have some provisions requiring written consent. Oklahoma, Kansas, Georgia, North Carolina, Texas and Connecticut require written consent from both the husband and wife. Arkansas and California require the written consent of the husband only.

Although the state of New York has passed no stature protecting the AID child, New York City has regulated the practice of AID through its Health Code since 1948. The ordinance provides that no donor shall have 'any disease or defect known to be transmissible by the genes.' It restricts the practice of artificial insemination to physicians, requires blood grouping and Rh typing of donors and calls for recording of the names and addresses of all donors (N.Y. City Health Code, art. 21, sect. 21.01-.07, 1959). The ordinance does not serve the function of legitimizing AID children; its purpose is to regulate AID practice from a public health standpoint.

In Georgia the child or children born of AID shall be considered by law in all respects the same as a naturally conceived child of the husband and wife consenting and requesting in writing the use of such technique (Behrman 1979). In Georgia, also, only practicing licensed physicians and surgeons are allowed to perform artificial insemination.

In Oklahoma, Kansas, California, Arkansas and North Carolina the AID child has been recognized specifically as either legitimate or entitled to the same rights as a naturally conceived child.

8. UNIFORM LEGISLATION

The US Uniform Parentage Act has a section specifically dealing with AID. Section 5a states that 'If, under the supervision of a licensed physician and with the consent of her husband, a wife is inseminated artificially with the sperm donated by a man not her husband, the husband is treated by law as the natural father of the child thereby conceived.' The husband's consent might be in writing and signed by him as well as his wife. The physician shall certify the signature and the date of insemination and file the husband's consent with the State Department of Health where it shall be kept confidential and in a sealed file. However the physician's failure to do so does not affect the father-child relationship. All papers and records pertaining to the insemination, whether part of the permanent record of the court or of the file held by the supervising physician or elsewhere, are subject to inspection only upon an order of the court for good cause shown.

Section 5b explains that the donor who provides sperm to a licensed physician for use in artificial insemination of a married woman other than the donor's wife is treated by law as if he were not the natural father of a child thereby conceived.

9. CONCLUDING REMARKS

In the final analysis one statement can be made with certainty about the present state laws regarding problems of AID: legislation is needed.

9.1. AID Legislation

The key question is whether, in the light of the world population explosion, AID legislation should be encouraged at all, allowing childless couples to bring children into the world. The answer is not apparent due to the absence of any correlative studies to indicate the relationship between existing AID statutes and their influence upon birth rates in the states that have enacted them. The absence of any empirical data to the contrary would seem to indicate that condoning AID via legislation would have no adverse effect on birth rates. A precise legal status for AID children would require legislation or judicial decision. There is at present a dearth of statutory law or case decisions to clarify that legal status.

New uniform legislation is needed to regulate the practice of AID and to define the rights and duties of the parties involved: the physician, recipient and her husband, the donor and his wife, as well as the AID child. These laws should:

1. Permit only physicians to administer artificial insemination – their specific duties should be defined;

2. Insure that the couple be properly evaluated by psychiatrists and social workers;
3. Require written consent of the recipient and her husband on a prescribed form;
4. Define specific guidelines for the selection of donors;
5. Obligate the donor to disclose, to the best of his knowlege, any history of physical, congenital and psychiatric illness of his own and/or his blood relatives;
6. Require a complete medical examination of the donor, and;
7. Specify that the donor and his wife sign a consent form permitting utilization of his sperm, surrendering any rights in relation to the child born of the insemination, and agreeing not to seek the identity of the recipient or the child. It must be made clear that the donor has no legal rights or obligations in respect to the child conceived from his sperm.

9.2. Precautionary measures

Meanwhile the physician practicing AID must take abundant precautions to obtain proper consent forms, signed by all parties involved. The general form book published by the Law Department of the American Medical Association includes three forms devoted to artificial insemination.

The first form is to be signed by the husband and wife before the wife undergoes artificial insemination. Its purpose is mainly to insure that:
1. The physician has made no guarantee;
2. The physician will not be liable for complications in childbirth or pregnancy or for the birth of an abnormal or hereditarily defective infant, and;
3. The physician will have the discretion to choose the donor and neither the husband nor the wife will seek to learn his identity.

The second form is signed by the donor, granting permission to use his sperm for possible impregnation of a direct recipient. The third form is signed only by the wife of the donor, in which she agrees to refrain from attempting to learn the identity of the recipient.

REFERENCES

Amelar RD, Dubin L, Gordan J, Tendler MD: Male infertility practice and orthodox Jewish law. *Urology* 10:177, 1977.
Beck WW Jr: A critical look at the legal, ethical and technical aspects of artificial insemination. *Fertil Steril* 27:1, 1976.
Behrman SJ: Artificial insemination and public policy. *New Engl J Med* 300:619, 1979.
Behrman SJ, Kistner RW: A rational approach to the evaluation of infertility. In: *Progress in infertility*. Behrman SJ, Kistner RW (eds), Boston. Little. Brown. 1968, p 1.

Carr JE: Artificial insemination: Problems, policies, and proposals. *Ala Law Rev* 26:120, 1973.

Curie-Cohen M, Luttrell L, Shapiro S: Current practice of artificial insemination by donor in the US. *New Engl J Med* 300:585, 1979.

Frankel MD: Artificial insemination: the medical profession and public policy. *Conn Med* 38:476, 1974.

Goldenberg RL, White R: Artificial insemination. *J Reprod Med* 18:149, 1977.

Healey JM Jr: Legal aspects of artificial insemination by donor and paternity testing. In: *Genetics and the law*, Milunsky A, Annas GJ (eds), New York, Plenum, 1976, p 203.

Kraus J: Expectancy of fertility after adoption. *Aust Soc Work* 29:19, 1976.

Kraus J, Quinn PE: Human artificial insemination: some social and legal issues. *Med J Aust* 1:710, 1977.

Macourt DC, Jones GR: Artificial insemination with donor semen. *Med J Aust* 1:693, 1977.

Rosenberg AH: Legal aspects of artificial insemination. *New Engl J Med* 278:552, 1968.

SUBJECT INDEX